Enactments

EDITED BY RICHARD SCHECHNER

To perform is to imagine, represent, live and enact present circumstances, past events and future possibilities. Performance takes place across a very broad range of venues from city streets to the countryside, in theatres and in offices, on battlefields and in hospital operating rooms. The genres of performance are many, from the arts to the myriad performances of everyday life, from courtrooms to legislative chambers, from theatres to wars to circuses.

ENACTMENTS will encompass performance in as many of its aspects and realities as there are authors able to write about them.

ENACTMENTS will include active scholarship, readable thought and engaged analysis across the broad spectrum of performance studies.

T03B5608

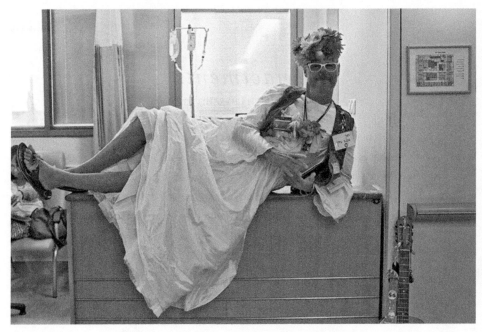

IMAGE 0.1 Amnon Raviv on duty. Rabin Medical Centre, Petach Tikva, 2015.
Photograph by Hazi Panet.

MEDICAL CLOWNING

THE HEALING PERFORMANCE

Amnon Raviv

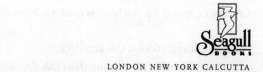

LONDON NEW YORK CALCUTTA

Seagull Books, 2018

Text © Amnon Raviv

Photographs © Individual photographers

Some photographs have been altered to protect patient privacy.

ISBN   978 0 8574 2 387 0

British Library Cataloguing-in-Publication Data

A catalogue record for this book is available from the British Library

Typeset by Seagull Books, Calcutta, India

Printed and bound by CPI Group (UK) Ltd, Croydon, CR0 4YY

*Dedicated with love
to my beloved children Toot and Yam
and my dear parents Esther and Tuvia.*

Contents

Acknowledgments

With special thanks to Prof. Richard Schechner, members of the Dream Doctors Project, Prof. Atay Citron, and to the amazing patients I met at the Department of Oncology, Chaim Sheba Medical Center, Tel HaShomer, Israel.

The Manifesto of the Order of the Red Nose

THE PROF. DR. DEPARTMENT HEAD

I hereby establish the Order of the Red Nose.

The goal of the Order is to create a more humane world.

To nullify the burdensome seriousness and replace it with light and lightening non-seriousness.

Members of the Order of the Red Nose shall operate as a "fifth column."

Their subversive activities shall be reflected through infiltration of all medical centers, hospitals, organizations, workplaces, offices, supermarkets, markets, clinics, public institutions, political parties, religious institutions, and houses of prayer. They shall disseminate the good news of levity to the cold and serious world in which we live.

The Order aims to cause irreversible damage, to be like a bug in the program of all institutions owning the narratives and the beliefs, overblown with their own importance and seriousness.

And to all economic, political, and religious institutions that use the same software of bottomless seriousness, and the aggressive and blind belief in the justice of any overweening pathway whatsoever.

Seriousness is frightening and fatal.

We shall now commence in gibberish. Too much seriousness is out of place.

Seriousness kills.

Let us move the center of gravity from seriousness to laughter.

Long live the Clownish Revolution!!!

We shall be right in a minority and in a minor way, therefore we shall not need to fight the "enemy," and shall have no need to redeem anyone. This is a paradoxical faith, convenient and user-friendly for the greater good of humankind.

Based on our experience over the past few millennia, the integration of art, craft, faith, and fundamentalism with total realism has not really worked.

On the contrary, it has proven itself to be most maleficent.

Instead, I propose the dawn of a new era: The Era of Power to the Red Nose!

I call upon you to join me. Life is a joke, so leave your synagogues, churches, monasteries, pagodas, huts, tents, igloos, projects housing, temples, offices, factories, plants, houses, army base, and workplaces, and join the Clown Army. Decorate your robes, skullcaps, suits, saris, top hats, keffiyehs, and veils in vibrant colors.

Wear the medals of seashells and flowers that you have made and given to yourselves and to others.

Laugh with an empathic laugh, since laughter liberates and a laugh is an embrace.

Prepare yourselves for the funeral of murderous seriousness.

Long live the clown's naivety!

Prepare thyself for the clown's clarion call: Fart, fart, fart . . . Long live the Red Nose!

And now, a few words, from our friends the Medical Clowns

The Medical Clown is a member of the Clown Family, a licensed idiot working toward the well-being of the patients and their families as well as of the ensemble of employees in the hospital.

Medical Clowns enact the utmost fantastic to build castles in the air. They strive to redress injustice and take over control of the government. They attempt to command armies, to make a huge impression with long speeches that have no particular message. They do their best to flatter and to avoid all responsibility.

Above all, they do their best to embrace the patients (mostly— but, not only—on a metaphorical level, of course, so as not to be infected by contagious diseases).

The Medical Clown will always strive to achieve the position of General Director of the Medical Center—or, at least, Head of the Department.

As a matter of principle, Medical Clowns deny all pain and ill-ness, and rashes and infections. They striving with all their might to be loved, to make people laugh, to create a bond, to make an impression, to reduce pain, to lower anxiety levels, to blow bubbles, write poems, fly through the air, set sail across the seas, provide ridiculous instructions, provide learned diagnoses, and/or dance, and perform the most splendid splits.

The Medical Clown is a living paradox who succeeds in not succeeding in a phenomenal way.

The Medical Clown is like a poet in nature, sensitive and emo-tional yet preferring to camouflage his feelings with crudity, to con-cealing his shyness with exaggerated extrovert behavior.

The Medical Clown takes no one and nothing into considera-tion. For example, if the Medical Clown spots a patient suffering from an illness, examination or procedure, he will always, always insist on starting a conversation on weird and wonderful topics, from the bizarre to the fantastical, from the unfounded to the delu-sional, acompanied by funny faces all the while.

Medical Clowns are self-appointed philosophers. They may, however, disguise themselves as a commandant or an expert on love.

They love honorifics, they are serially insulted; they are always in love, and they are always full of enthusiasm.

They pretend to be linguists and are multitalented.

The Medical Clown is also a witness. He can give evidence of anxiety, suffering, joy, hope, unconsciousness, hopelessness, recovery, fatigue. He can testify about patients, paraprofessionals, therapists, helpless parents, hospital childhoods, old age, and oblivion, despair, alienation, acceptance, humanity, love, strength and weakness.

He can also testify about devotion, abandonment, tears, laughter, foolishness, wisdom, appreciation, crudity, rudeness, and pain. It's all there, in the hospital.

The Medical Clown can testify to recovery.

The Medical Clown can testify to a short, gentle life that fades out.

The Medical Clown can testify to a short life that terminated in suffering.

The Medical Clown belongs to the Family of Clowns who are idiots licensed for the general public, for "everyone."

The Medical Clown has idiotic questions for the Lord too.

CHAPTER ONE

Still the Best Medicine, Even in a War Zone
My Work as a Medical Clown

Who and what is a clown doctor? Is he or she an artist of emotions, or some sort of performer/therapist?

Medical clowning has increased in prominence over the past 20 years; and, over the past 10 especially, been used in treating Post-Traumatic Stress Disorder (PTSD) for people in war zones and in the wake of natural disasters.

The modern medical clown stems from two roots: the first, clowning, from street performers to court jesters and kings' fools to theatrical and circus clowns; the second, the figure of the healer, the shaman, and the witch doctor. Indeed, medical clowns have been called "the shaman healers of Western medicine" (Van Blerkom 1995: 462).

Unlike the more familiar clown figure, whose task through history has been to critique social and political ills, the task of the medical clown is to assist in the healing process of patients in medical centers and convalescent homes. This the medical clown does by employing humor and fantasy and creating an alternative world, a world radically different from the immediate reality of the ailing or suffering person. Encouraging an awareness and experience of the vital life force within the patient, medical clowns significantly reduce anxiety among the institutionalized, especially trauma victims, and thus accelerate the healing process.

My work as a medical clown has been with shock victims at Barzilai Medical Center, Ashkelon, southern Israel, as part of the Dream Doctors Project[1] founded by the Philnor Foundation. When I began this work, I was already an experienced theater practitioner,

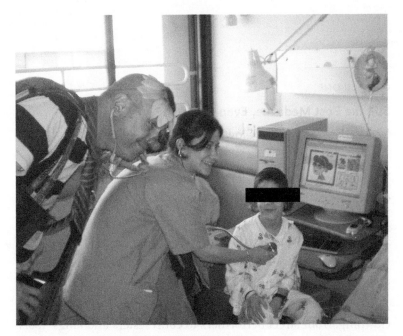

FIGURE 1.1 The medical clown sometimes checks the doctor the same way the doctor checks the patient. Chaim Sheba Medical Center, Tel HaShomer, 2011.

and a teacher in the Theater Department at Haifa University. Here I will concentrate on my work as a medical clown during the three weeks of the War in Gaza—"Operation Cast Lead"[2]—that took place from late December 2008 to January 2009.

Humor and laughter are the tools of the medical clown. But do these really help patients to recover? Vera M. Robinson in *Humor and the Health Professions* (1991) described laughter as a weapon to help us cope with existence. In Freudian terms, reality tends to repress the ego while humor releases it. Robinson considered the physiological research on the effects of humor, its biochemical impact, and the association of humor with the cognitive emotional system a unique psychophysical phenomena. Humor stimulates laughter, a forceful series of bursts of breath and sound that increase the heartbeat and oxygen flow to the brain, release endorphins, and strengthen the immune system.

A hearty laugh also results in muscle relaxation and emotional release. According to Raymond A. Moody in *Laugh After Laugh: The Healing Power of Humor* (1978), a sense of humor requires the ability to look at oneself and the world from a disconnected viewpoint, the ability to gazie on existence from an alternate perspective. Such a position not only makes laughter possible but also allows for a positive emotional involvement with people and events.

The medical clown offers a patient precisely such a perspective, and thereby ways with which to cope with stress and anxiety. In a film created by the Philnor Foundation in 2009, Dr. Ron Lobel, deputy director of Barzilai Medical Center, states, "Laughter and humor have a very important function in the stages of healing of all internal disease. We know that they assist in the secretion of endorphins, the hormones with a positive impact on the healing processes for most illnesses" In the same film, Prof. Francis Maimoni, director of the pediatrics unit at Shaare Zedek Medical Center, Jerusalem, says, "The clown-doctor comes over to the patient to heal as I attempt to heal, but we each use different tools. The medical clown captures the patient's attention, bringing him into another world which does not exist within the hospital walls."

Patients can feel all to easily that they are on the lowest rung of the hospital's alienating structure, with its physicians at the top, then the nurses and then all the other personnel. The overwhelming layout of such institutions, often with their many rooms and corridors, as well as all the intimidating equipment, can increase the patient's trepidation. So it is equally important that a medical clown uses his sense of humor to also seemingly strike a blow at a hospital's hierarchy and its anxiety-producing routines.

I have recorded in my diary some moments of my work with Prof. Menahem Shlezinger, former head of pediatrics at Barzilai Medical Center. We would, for example, duel with my sponge swords along the corridors and in the rooms, taking some doctors and nurses "hostage" and trying to recruit young patients to our side. The kids (who would go wild with laughter) were then allowed to name the winner. The honorable professor was as enthusiastic as the kids, a great collaborator and an inspiration to the other medical staff. By introducing such a carnival spirit and prompting outbursts of derisive laughter, the clown upturns the hospital's rigid social structure which in turn helps restore a sense of control to the patient and, moreover, helps the staff release their own stress.

The catharsis generated by the medical clown thus differs from the catharsis provided by classical theater. The Aristotelian notion of catharsis is possible when events do not directly affect the observer. In contrast, the catharsis of a patient interacting with a medical clown is more intimate, and uses a different kind of distance than that about which Aristotle theorizes. The patient cannot distance the threat within their own body, but, helped by the medical clown, they can assume a different viewpoint and use their laughter to stimulate the life force within them, the will to help them to survive life-threatening situations.

Paul McGhee cites an important piece of research on cancer patients that took place over seven years in Norway: "Those scoring higher on a sense of humor test at the beginning of the study had a 70 per cent higher survival rate than those with a poorer sense of humor" (2010: 213). And in her research on humor in the Holocaust, Chaya Ostrower quotes survivors discussing their terrible experiences: "If not for humor we would have committed suicide"; "Humor is one of the ingredients of the mental strength and the will to live"; "Humor is an inner command to survive" (2009: 69, 57, 73; all translations from Hebrew are my own).

One day at the hospital, I entered a room in which all four beds were concealed behind closed curtains. I made a few funny noises and asked for permission to open the curtains. The kids in the beds were of different ages, and they all had family members sitting beside them. The harsh glare of the neon lights tinged all their faces with gray; the kid on the bed in the left corner looked especially pale and his mother, very tense.

"Hello everybody," I began, "welcome to our hotel. Breakfast will be served soon. Here, in the meantime, is our Jacuzzi" (*I pointed to the sink*). "And there, through the window, you can see the famous Mont Blanc and the beautiful Alps (*I pointed to the window in the corridor*). And you can breathe in the fresh and healthy air."

Then I began to mumble absurdly in a French accent and performed some tricks. And I danced and sang a song in Russian about the famous cosmonaut Yuri Gagarin.

The mother on the left—the one who had been so tense— suddenly burst into peals of laughter. It was a laugh that released all her anxiety and there was nothing she could do to stop it.

I was very "angry" with her and tried to make her stop. But the more I tried, the more she laughed. I even sprinkled water on her, but it only made it worse.

FIGURE 1.2 Amnon Raviv with Dr. Ron Lobel, Deputy Director, Barzilai Medical Center, Ashkelon, 2009.

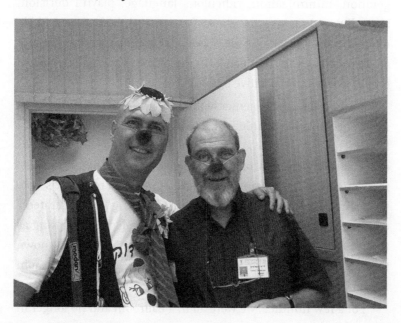

Laughter is contagious, and before long, everyone in the room was exploding with laughter. Some people strolled over from the next room to see what was going on. I began to "worry" about the mother and shouted to a nurse to come quickly. Dalia, the nurse, rushed in. "What happened?!" she asked. When I explained, she said, "Don't shout like that, I was really alarmed!" But she relaxed when I told her I was in love with her—I got down on my knees and gave her a plastic flower.

By the time I moved on to the next room, they were all smiling as they waved farewell and blew kisses at me.

The medical clown's presence and the playfulness they bring to the hospital can create social connections that transcend the constricted space and the lack of privacy. The clown helps patients and their families shatter emotional barriers so that they can share their feelings and empathize with one another.

With comic theatrical strategies, such as the turnaround, exaggeration, minimization, ridiculous language, playful derision, absurdity, and fantasy, the clown "transports" the patient outside of the medical center, outside of everyday concerns and worries, to an alternative "site" that can help the patient experience medical events with a more positive outlook.

For example, in the center of the pediatric unit at Barzilai Medical Center there is a little hall. It was never meant to be a space for patients but space was scarce. One morning I decided that this space could become a ballroom. I gave the kids small musical instruments to accompany my singing. I invited a nurse, Iris, into the ballroom to dance with me. Before dancing, I exaggeratedly confessed that I was in love with her. The kids were giggling as they started to play. The Iris and I danced while I sang well-known tunes with gibberish words. Soon after, I made all the parents join in and dance as couples with others.

For a few minutes, we were all in a ballroom and no longer in a hospital.

The medical clown's job is to disrupt the seriousness of the medical regimen and thus, paradoxically, enhance the effectiveness of treatment. Here are two examples of constructive disruption:

When I take part in a medical procedure, I sometimes examine a doctor in the same way in which they examine a patient. From the kid's point of view, the procedure becomes a sort of game, and they are more relaxed and the treatment, therefore, more effective.

I also work with adult patients in the dialysis ward at Hartzfeld Hospital in Gedera. One morning I was told by the nurse that, a few minutes before my arrival, an elderly patient, a double amputee (he had lost both his legs) had been in a terrible rage, cursing and trying to hit the nurses. He had been so violent that they had even called for the police. I looked at him, and I made a quick "diag-red-nosis"—I noticed the big kippah (a yarmulke) on his head, so I took my guitar and began to sing a famous song from the Psalms. He began to sing with me, and then, slowly, to smile. Out of the corner of my eye I saw three policemen talking to the nurse . . . and then leave. In the middle of what could have been an extreme incident, I caused a disruption and made the resumption of medical routine possible.

Medical clowning is a site-specific performance that transforms the space in which it takes place—the hospital is no longer a formidable locus of paraphernalia and uniformed staff but a place of fantasy created and shared by clown and patient.

One such transformation took place at the pediatrics unit of Barzilai, in Room No. 5, the room for children who suffer from contagious illnesses. Transparent dividers separated the beds. As soon as I stepped into the room, it became a big aquarium. I blew soap bubbles as if they are underwater air bubbles; I imitated sea creatures as I got closer to the transparent dividers and looked at the kids, in the same way as fish in the aquarium look at visitors through the glass of their tanks.

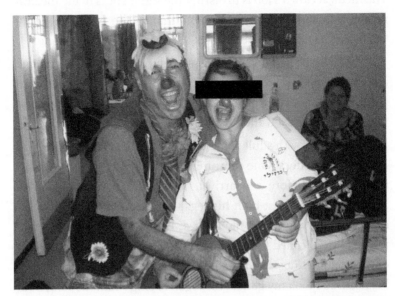

FIGURE 1.3 (ABOVE). The clown transports the patient outside of the medical center, sometimes by making them a part of the show. Barzilai Medical Center, Ashkelon, 2008.

FIGURE 1.4 (BELOW). Physical pain can be reduced by dissociating the patient from their immediate situation. Chaim Sheba Medical Center, Tel HaShomer, 2011.

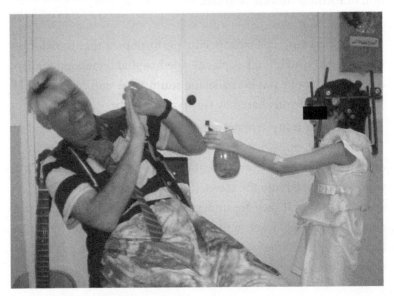

In another fantasy world, I sometimes transform the long corridors of the pediatric ward in Chaim Sheba Medical Center into skiing lanes. I hold my sponge swords as if they are ski poles, put on my sunglasses, and glide with the kids on imaginary skis.

The medical clown works with three circles of audiences: at the center are the hospitalized; then, the patient's family and friends; and finally, the hospital staff. Sometimes alleviating the parents' anxiety, eliciting a smile from them, has an immediate impact on a child's condition. At other times, working with the parents is a tactic to reach the child. The clown is also an integral member of the staff, not only working with them but also providing them with much needed comic relief.

Like the shaman, the medical clown transports their patients. In "Clown Doctors: Shaman Healers of Western Medicine," Linda Miller Van Blerkom notes that both the shaman and the medical clown develop alternative, believed-in realities (1995). Michael Harner describes the shaman as entering an alternate state of consciousness, bringing others along with him with the intention of healing. This is exactly what the medical clown does. Milton Erickson in *The Nature of Hypnosis and Suggestion* (1980) discusses the perception of another reality generated by the power of suggestion, and proposes that both ways of understanding reality (with and without suggestion) can exist simultaneously. In such a case, a person chooses the alternative reality in order to meet the needs created by circumstances. Erickson says that physical pain can be reduced by separating the person from their immediate situation.

It is pertinent at this point to refer to John Shea's description of pain reduction through both auto- and external suggestion by stating that the placebo effect is evidence of human beings' inherent capacity for self-healing through suggestion (1991). Shea cites research studies that have found organic changes in the bloodstream and brain cells induced through suggestion. One such experience was reported in the newspapers: Omer was a 9-year-old girl with a chronic disease that required regular, painful treatments. She would make her appointment on a day when she knew I would be working at the pediatric outpatient clinic. And she refused to have anyone but me accompany her to the treatment room, not even her mother. On our way to the treatment room, we would perform a wild dance and sing, a rap we'd written together about all the characters involved in the medical procedures: Omer, the clown (me), Omer's mother, and Riva, the nurse. The refrain was "there will be no pain." It is precisely this ritual song-and-dance that imbued Omer with the strength to withstand her painful procedures.

Young children, especially, believe in the medical clown's powers and remedies: invisible magic powders, spells, and rituals conjured by the clown. I have lessened pain with an invisible powder sprinkled on many a young patient. One kind of invisible powder is in the sunflower in my head; another is in the sunflower on my vest. Before I show a child the right way to mix them, I need to check their magical abilities. This I do with my magic book whose pages are ordinarily blank and will reveal pictures only if the person who touches them has magic powers. How happy I am to find a child with such magic powers! We mix the invisible powders and then, whispering spells in gibberish, I sprinkle it on the pain. The interesting thing about this ritual is that, according to the kids, it helps, even though some of them know that it is not "real."

Treating PTSD

Ever since July 8, 2004, my very first day as a medical clown (with the Dream Doctors Project), I have worked with trauma patients. I worked with them during the nightmarish years of 2004 until the end of 2008, until the onset of Operation Cast Lead. The residents of the southern Israeli town of Sderot and the comunities of Gaza Envelope were under constant attack from the Gaza Strip. Thousands of mortar shells and Qassam rockets landed on the Israelis, destroying homes and injuring and killing residents. Just as damaging as the mayhem was the trauma this barrage had caused.

At 7:38 a.m. on Monday, September 3, 2007, a Qassam rocket fell on Sderot, narrowly missing a schoolbus carrying 35 elementary-school children. The stunned children were rushed to Barzilai and then into the hospital's dining room, the only room large enough to hold them all together. There the children were met by a professional team of psychologists, psychiatrists, social workers, physicians, and nurses.

I was at the hospital that morning and heard purely by chance about what had happened.

As I rushed toward the dining room, one of the psychologists gestured to me, trying to say: "It's not a good time now." But I felt that it was exactly the right time for a clown.

I went in, and as is proper for a clown (an undisciplined creature with no sense of boundaries), I sat down among the children seated in a circle of chairs. The children were pale and withdrawn. The psychologist who had not wanted me there was talking, but were the children listening?

As I sat down, my bag "accidentally" opened, and all my clowning stuff fell out. I apologized, made faces, gathered everything, and checked all my gadgets to make sure they still worked. The children began to laugh. Within a few minutes, their pale faces brightened up and some of their anxiety and shock began to dissipate.

I stayed with the children even while they were being examined by the staff. As we went from station to station, hand in hand, we pretended we were in an imaginary forest. Then it was lunchtime. We all sat down to eat, and very quickly, the meal became a food fight and the children were overcome with laughter.

Dr. Ron Lobel and Dr. Emile Hay, deputy directors of the hospital, told us that our work that day had made a deep impression on them.

After this incident, the three medical clowns working in Barzilai (Hagar Hofesh, Jerome Harosh, and I) began to receive more encouragement from the hospital administration. All of us were part of the Dream Doctors Project. We worked separately, for three hours every morning on different days, but in emergencies we worked much longer. At 6 p.m. on May 14, 2008, a Katyusha-Grad rocket launched from the northern Gaza Strip near Beit Lahiya landed in the crowded Hutzot Mall in Ashkelon. Fifteen people were injured, four seriously and eleven moderately. Sixty-two traumatized people were immediately evacuated to Barzilai.

During the rest of the day, the numbers of those with shock trauma continued to rise.

The hospital administrators summoned the clowns at once. Over the next few days we made many calls to the various departments working with the traumatized patients. Every time I was called, I packed up my Stress Treatment Kit—a collection of tools and strange objects I had gathered to help me "disperse" stress and "exorcize" fears: clean wrap to protect against missiles; kitchen utensils to massage with; a flashlight to use as a microphone; a safety pin to hold positive thoughts in place; a flyswatter to stimulated circulation; etc.

When I discovered that some of the injured wanted to talk about their experiences, I "interviewed" them by pretending to be a reporter from a TV station in India, with a lead-in of Bollywood dancers and, as a break during the interview, a traditional Indian song.

I also attempted to "sell" my special "Personal Protective Security Kit," with the clean wrap stretched out toward the Gaza Strip to hold back the Katyusha rockets. The absurdity of the flimsy barrier made people laugh, but no less importantly it helped them let off steam. Criticism and juicy curses lambasted the government for failing to provide enough security shelters for the residents of the communities near Gaza.

During the War in Gaza (Operation Cast Lead), which lasted from December 29, 2008 to January 15, 2009, the three of us

Dream Doctors divided up the shifts, each of us working alone. I put in long shifts at the emergency room at Barzilai Medical Center (partially security reinforced).

One day, a barrage of Qassam rockets fell on the town, some raining down on the hospital grounds and others on the street where I live. My trip to the hospital usually takes only a few minutes; but that day it became a long journey interrupted by several red alerts. I had to stop my car and lie on the ground until the rockets hit. When I finally arrived at the hospital, I found an emergency room full of shock victims. Dozens after dozens would come in during the three weeks of the war.

In what was perhaps one of my most difficult cases, a trauma victim was trembling violently, incapable of hearing a word I said. And it was only after she received a sedative injection, that I was able to work with her. She was a young woman, around 25 years old, accompanied by her fiancé and her parents. Her fiancé mentioned that they planned to get married in two months. So I said to all of them, "Listen, I am going to give you a demonstration of the wedding—all you have to do is to put names to the characters I'll show you." Then I started to mime grotesque parodies of different people eating, walking, dancing, talking, etc. And they were delighted: "This one walks like Uncle Simon, and this one eats like Aunty Freda . . . " and so on. Soon the fiancé and the parents were laughing, but not the patient. So I announced that the time had come for the newly married couple to dance, and started to dance with the fiancé as if I was the bride. I did it in such an exaggerated and funny way that it was only a few moments before a big smile spread across her face, and I knew that she was "back."

The psychologist and nurse who had asked me to work with the young woman were also doubled over with laughter. This act of clowning helped them too, tense and fatigued that they were and anxious about their families back home. After each rocket fell, they rushed to phone home and check that everyone was all right.

We worked very closely with the staff who sometimes laughed even more than the patients. And I never heard any complaints that we were disrupting their work.

I spent New Year's Day 2009, in the emergency room of Barzilai Medical Center. Rockets fell every few minutes. Many of those streaming into the E.R. were injured, but the majority were trauma victims. I was appointed to admit those in shock for "primary care" and took time between patients to treat the staff.

Shortly after one of the Qassam rockets fell in a heavily populated area of town, a family stumbled in. A rocket had exploded only a few meters away from them. They were all traumatized: a girl, about 10 years old, was screaming in fear; her mother and grandmother were crying, and her father was pale and silent.

I led them to a quiet corner and began treating them all simultaneously. I demonstrated some magic tricks to the girl (I will call her Dana), and introduced her to Madame Esther, my finger puppet. Madame Esther is a former world and Olympic champion in gymnastics and swimming. Willing to show Dana some of her amazing abilities, she performed a hand-stand, then balanced on her nose, then jumped into the pool and began to swim.

I gave an "anti-worry" massage to the grandmother with my kitchen implements and flyswatter. I pampered the father with a hairstyle and haircut, pretending to trim the hair from his nostrils and ears. I also made sure to provide a soapy anti-dandruff shampoo, complete with "straightening treatment" from a "hairdryer" (I requested a passing security guard to blow air on the nostrils).

Finally, little Dana began to laugh and helped me style her father's nose hair.

Dana's laughter, and my antics, also managed to calm the mother, and slowly, she began to smile too. By the time I finished, the family was feeling a lot more secure. I wrote a hospital discharge letter for them, including a prescription for a menu full of rich and varied delicacies and all sorts of special desserts, and Viagra for the father because stress is known to destroy performance. The father laughed good-naturedly, the mother nodded her approval, and the grandmother had no idea what it was all about.

Dana, who had been hysterical when she arrived, happily waved goodbye and blew me a kiss.

I pulled myself together and geared up for the next group of trauma victims. But first I phoned my kids to make sure everything was OK. "Yes, Dad, we're fine. A rocket fell on our street, not far from the house. Sure we heard the big explosion, unbelievable! But we're fine, don't worry . . . "

Notes

1   The Dream Doctors Project integrates professional medical clowning into the medical services provided at Israeli hospitals. Established in 2002, the Dream Doctors Project is now operating in 18 hospitals throughout the country, with 72 medical clowns working in various pediatric wards and clinics. The project aims to develop clowning therapy by promoting academic research in this field and establishing a professional community. Toward this aim, a unique bachelor's program in clowning therapy has been created at Haifa University. The program is currently expanding into a master's degree.

Dream Doctors operate in internal care, surgery, intensive care, operating rooms, outpatient clinics, diabetes clinics, HIV-AIDS clinics, external care, rehabilitation, dialysis, daycare centers for autistic children, oncology units, neonatal and premature baby wards, centers for child victims of sexual abuse, and psychiatric wards.

Dream Doctors play a unique role in facilitating cross-cultural liaisons across religious, ethnic, and national lines. Their expressive abilities enable them to bridge opposites, calm fears, and inspire trust in the medical team and the treatment process. It is quite often impossible to treat certain children without the presence of a Dream Doctor who mediates between the patients and the "white jackets."

The Dream Doctors Project was established and operates under the sponsorship of the Philnor Foundation (a registered non-profit association). For more information on the project and its initiatives, please visit http://dreamdoctors.org.il/en/ (last accessed on May 15, 2017).

2 Over those years, Hamas launched thousands of missiles and rockets into southern Israel. In retaliation, Israel invaded Gaza in an operation called Operation Cast Lead. As a medical clown, I encountered dozens of children and adults (Israelis and Palestinians) hospitalized with Acute Stress Disorder (ASD) and Post-Traumatic Stress Disorder (PTSD).

CHAPTER TWO

Clowning to Death

My Work as a Medical Clown with Terminally Ill Patients

Medical clowning is a flexible performance that needs to be calibrated according to the patient's age, personality, and state of health in order to reduce the anxiety of impending death for both the patient and their family.

In this chapter, I will attempt to describe and analyze six case studies with terminally ill patients. Five took place with adult patients and their families in various departments of a medical center while the sixth was an encounter with an ill child at his home.

Medical clowning in public hospitals began in 1986 in New York City as part of the Big Apple Circus Clown Care Unit program, formulated by Michael Christensen in association with Infants and Children's Hospital (Citron 2011; Pendzik and Raviv 2012a). Subsequently, additional programs began in hospitals around the world. Most medical clowns work with children in various pediatric units—children have a natural connection to clowns, for they represent the world of the imagination. In recognition of this connection, hospitals almost everywhere are willing to open their gates to the clowns and their paraphernalia and their spirit of jesting and laughter.

In recent years, I have been working with adult oncology patients in Chaim Sheba Medical Center at Tel HaShomer, not far from Tel Aviv, and with the chronically ill at Hartzfeld Hospital, Gedera.

But what is the nature of the medical clown's performance in the context of impending death? What makes it unique?

The Background

The healers of the !kung tribe and the witch doctors of the Azande care for the ill through a healing performance that mediates between the patient and the otherwise-inaccessible metaphysical world (the world of spirits and magic; see Evans-Pritchard 1976 and Shostak 1981). The medical clown has been called a modern shaman (Van Blerkom 1995) who, like these traditional healers, mediates between the hospitalized patient and the world of fantasy, carnival spirit, and humor, thereby helping the terminally ill to cope with their illness, fears, and uncertainties.

The following stories show how each of the patients I have worked with had a different need and thus required a singular clowning performance, directly resulting from his personality and the unique interaction between us. The first three case studies are about my clowning performance with adult terminally ill patients in the Oncology Department of Chaim Sheba Medical Center. The fourth and fifth are about my clowning performances with adult patients who passed away (or more correctly, with the people who accompanied the late patient) at Hartzfeld Geriatric Hospital (one passed away during a performance in the dialysis room). The sixth is about a child with cancer, my clowning performance at his house, and the deep sadness I experienced after he passed away.

The "Carnivalesque"

Rina [a pseudonym, as are all the names in this chapter] was a woman in her 50s or 60s, whose condition was deteriorating rapidly. Entering her room, over the few months that I visited her, I would begin to dance wildly to music blaring from my small tape recorder, accompanied by her two sons and husband.

Rina would stare at us with a severe expression, and make sharp comments about my sense of rhythm and choreography. For, despite the cancer in her head, she had lost neither her dry sense of humor nor her cynicism. But, without a doubt, the more wilder our dance became, the more pleased she was.

Sometimes I would sing songs of her choosing, accompanying myself on my guitar—but in a grotesque parody. And she would look at me with both seriousness and amusement.

The last time we met, she was dying. Her husband asked me to hurry over. In the small room reserved for the dying, Rina lay in bed, eyes closed, surrounded by family. One of her sons held her hand, and with tears rolling down his face, he spoke to her softly and told her how much they all loved her.

Suddenly Rina opened her eyes. "You're making a hole in my head," she said to her son. Then, looking around at the rest of the famly, she said, "Oh ho, it doesn't look so good!" Everyone froze and looked down at their feet.

"Does this look better?" I asked, and broke out into a gig, dragging her husband and some of the other relatives into a last wild dance.

Rina nodded. "Better," she whispered, with a hint of a smile. Then she closed her eyes.

The carnivalesque is the human being's emotional and physical resistance to repression (Fiske 1989b). Clowns have, through history, enflamed and increased the people's carnivalesque expressions of opposition during annual celebrations and fairs. As Mikhail M. Bakhtin notes, the carnivalesque expresses not only objection to social repression but also reflects opposition to the existential state of human life; it is protest against the repression of life that produces illness and Death (1984).

Rina, with her strong, cynical personality, expressed a carnivalesque opposition to her condition and impending death. She scorned her illness and, in Allen Klein's words, addressed fear like a bullfighter in an arena (1998). And she used my clown-ish assistance to amplify the expression of that carnivalesque opposition. She was not sentimental, because there are no sentiments in war. It would be a mistake to assume that when she saw her dear ones around her bedside she understood it was the end—she had understood that a long time before. Rather, she wanted those around her to mirror her emotions, especially her opposition to the idea of a gloomy death. Carnivalesque laughter is what enables people to overcome the fear of death (ibid.), not only for the patient but also for the family.

Humor

I met Josef at the oncology day care unit at Chaim Sheba Medical Center. One day, I don't remember why, he changed his hospital schedule to coincide with one of my two working days there. Since then, Josef made sure to come in for treatment on the days I was present, so that we could meet. Every time he heard me approaching, he'd yell, "Here comes my buddy." Many of our jokes referred to his condition. One morning, a film crew came in to make a promotional film for the hospital. We "clowned around" for them and sang together as if we were in a Hollywood musical. Josef said that unlike the musicals, there would be no "happy end" here, and we both laughed. He loved to tell me about his life, and I would act out the major figures from his stories while he would burst out laughing.

Over time, his condition gradually deteriorated until he was hospitalized in the oncology ward.

The last time I saw him, we spoke thus:

ME. *Buongiorno*, Josef. How are you?

JOSEF. Soon I won't be farting anymore.

ME. It's about time. Everyone here is suffering from it.

JOSEF. Yes, but my kids are already used to the smell . . .

ME. They're suffering, too.

JOSEF. OK, well, at least I'm leaving them some money, and "money has no smell."

ME. I have a joke about farts . . .

JOSEF. They've told me that I'm terminal and suggested I
move to the hospice . . .

ME. Wow! It's like a hotel suite there, that's good.

JOSEF. Yeah, I heard there's a garden.

ME. I don't want to let you go until you bring me all of your
medical "grass" that you promised me.

JOSEF. Forget it, I'll need every gram.

ME. Oh, Josef, we had some good times . . . Do you remember when we appeared together in that film?

JOSEF. Yeah, and we were fantasizing about Hollywood . . .
Well, would you sing me a song? But not a lullaby . . .

ME. Are you nuts? You want me to get you to sleep and
then be accused of euthanasia?

JOSEF. Maybe that song by Louis Armstrong, "What a wonderful world?"

ME. I'd like to compose a song in your honor (*I begin to play
the instrument and sing*). Josef, you're a special wonderful man . . . a world-class farter . . . I love you . . .

JOSEF. I love you too, man. I bonded with you immediately.

ME. So you won't make it to your 120th birthday (*A traditional Jewish biblical anecdote that the maximum possible
age of a human being is 120 years, and is one of the most
common birthday blessings—"May you reach 120!"*)

JOSEF. No, I won't reach 120, but I'm satisfied that what I
did reach—. It is also something.

ME. It is quite something. Goodbye, Josef.

JOSEF. Goodbye.

A sense of humor requires the capacity to look at oneself and the
world in a somewhat detached and distanced manner, with a view
of reality that is objective rather than the terminally ill patient's

immediate, frightening, subjective one. Humor was Josef's existential choice in order to experience in an easier and less threatening manner the reality into which he was thrust.

Josef (like Rina), designed my clowning performance and the nature of our interaction according to his needs. In our last conversation, he hilariously describes himself as someone about to cease farting—a description of imminent death put forth in the most amusing and least frightening way. Josef said farewell with a smile, at peace with himself and the world. Democritus, "the laughing philosopher," observed that philosophy's final word on life was laughter.

It seems to me that Josef's laughter is the joyfulness which characterized him.

Fantasy

I met Haim many months before his passing. His parents had immigrated to Israel from Hungary, and he used to laugh at my descriptions of how I had learnt my broken Hungarian from the beautiful girlfriend I lived with on Rakocki Street in Budapest. I would mimic our "language lessons"—which took place in the bedroom—as a series of the moans and groans of lovemaking. Haim was curious to hear more about my life, so I spun him a fantasy, peppered with the odd grain of truth. He joined in my fantastical "biography" with his own special concoction of fact and fiction. Once he asked me how I made my living, so I told him I was a "gray market" moneylender and money changer; then I took out a roll of bills from my pocket and offered him a loan. Another time I told him my family owned a factory manufacturing digital and hydraulic valves for export to Singapore and Japan (with endless details on the structure and function of the valve) and that I was the plant manager. Everything was, of course, accompanied by grotesque clowning. I told him about my girlfriends in every port in every corner of the world, and Haim sailed away with me into the land of imagination and humor, far from the hospital ward, in an attempt to trace the truth in my stories which so amused him.

I did not have a chance to say goodbye to Haim. One morning Nurse Penina called me over and said that Haim had passed away, and that his wife Nina wanted to thank everyone, especially me. Later, I received an e-mail from Nina in which she wrote: "My smile is both sad and happy. Sad because my husband passed away, and happy because I discovered that there are wonderful people like you who can help by raising our spirits for a few moments. Sending you a huge hug, and I'm sure Haim sends one too—you knew how to make him laugh and give him some happiness."

The imagination has powers to heal the soul (Lahad 1992). Together, Haim and I, we traveled far from the oncology day unit to somewhere beyond time and place. Places, loves, and events melded together as we became young and beautiful and conquered the world. Fantasy enables us to enter worlds of never-ending possibilities. At the very heart of fantasy are relations between the human being and Eternity (Mathews 2002). The fantastic facilitates a dialogue with what is illogical and inexplicable in our lives (Pendzik and Raviv 2011). There was nothing logical about the illness that struck Haim in the middle of his life, a married man with two young children at home. The fantasy I invented for him, and in which he became a participant, helped him conduct an indirect conversation with his situation and his impending death.

"Extreme Clowning"

Hartzfeld Hospital's dialysis unit comprises two rooms. In the large room, dozens of patients are seated on armchairs and connected to dialysis machines. That morning, I was dancing with one of the nurses in front of the amused patients when Danny (a patient of about 70) began to wheeze loudly. The doctor and nurses hurried over and tried to help but the sounds ceased and so they called the resuscitation team. Despite the latter's attempts, there was nothing left but to declare Danny dead—the nurses covered his body, lying there in the armchair, with a sheet.

A man in his 60s, in the next chair, began to cry soundlessly, tears running down his face. Nurse Galit went over to him, patted his hand and tried to calm him. I was still reeling from the drama of the attempted resuscitation. The tears of Danny's neighbor cut into my reverie and prompted me to leave; clowning was perhaps not the most appropriate response in that difficult situation.

But Nurse Galit asked me to continue my performance—in her opinion, the patients needed me, their clown, now more than ever. So I resumed my jokes, all the anecdotes that I had ever known about dying and going to Heaven. The patient near Danny's chair slowly began to smile even as the tears coursed down his cheeks.

For months afterward, I had doubts about whether I had done the right thing by responding to the nurse's request to remain in the room, even though my instincts had urged me to leave. Had my performance and jokes really been suitable in those painful circumstances? I asked myself such questions until, finally, "the penny dropped" and I realized why this case was different from the others. So far, I had been invited either by the patient or their family to be present during the final moments of their dear ones and, at times, even after (as you will see in the next story). I would never have been present, nor performed, without such an invitation. A clowning performance at such a difficult time is not wanted by all patients or by all families. But in this case, Danny's death was public—not an intimate familial event. Was the clowning performance, therefore, able to dissipate or diminish the shock experienced by the others in the room? The nurse's opinion was "yes"—but I remained doubtful.

Ritual

Department E in Hartzfeld Hospital is the geriatric ward, the "last stop" for many of the patients. Some are hospitalized for a few days;

others remain for years before their souls return to the Creator; a very small fraction succeed in going back home.

One morning, while I performed in the ward lobby before several elderly patients, I heard someone crying and a commotion in one of the rooms. An old man had passed away. Two middle-aged women came out of the room (the man's daughters) and asked me to come into their father's room, where the body was lying, having been declared dead only moments before. I stood before the bed, without understanding why they had asked me in. The daughters were sobbing, begging me to do something. What did they mean? What was I supposed to do? They continued to cry, expecting me to take action. Finally, I began to strum my guitar and sing a quiet farewell song, composed on the spot, for a dead man I did not know, a man who lay in front of me, his eyes open, as I stood next to his weeping daughters.

When I think of the daughters' plea to "do something," I realize that the medical clown is a liminal figure who simultaneously belongs and does not belong to the hospital paradigm. He is part of and not a part of the medical team, entirely different in every aspect, from his costume to his medical responsibility. He "lands" in the hospital from the parallel reality of the imagination and humor, which differs from, and is alien to, the lived experience of the patients and their families. As a liminal figure, the medical clown is able to expand and empower what Richard Schechner has called the actual and conceptual space (2002). And this is precisely why the dead man's daughters decided to ask me to "do something." They chose a medical clown with the capacity to "move" between realities to mediate between them and their new reality of bereavement, a new reality that they felt was inaccessible to them. The "something" they asked for, as I understood it, was some kind of a farewell ritual. Don Handelman characterizes the ritualistic clown as a figure of paradox who facilitates the transition into the alternate experience of a ritual (1981). It may perhaps be possible for us to characterize the medical clown as a ritualistic figure as well. The farewell song that I composed and sang apparently

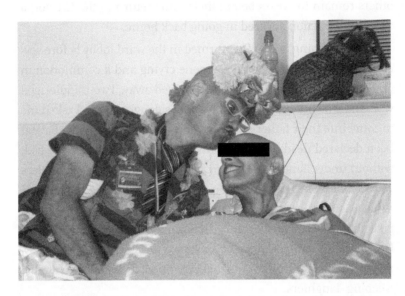

FIGURE 2.1 (ABOVE). A patient with the medical clown. Rabin Medical Center, Petach Tikva, 2015.

FIGURE 2.2 (BELOW). A patient with the medical clown. Chaim Sheba Medical Center, Tel HaShomer, 2012.

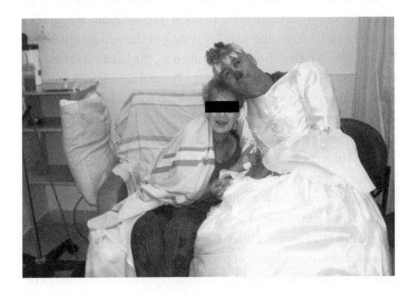

fulfilled the bereaved daughters' need for a ceremonial and personal farewell to their father.

The Birthday Party

My final story is about saying goodbye to a child. A friend of mine asked if I could visit a boy at home; he had been in her son's class, and the parents had asked her if I could visit. After three years of battling the disease, his doctors had given up and released the boy to spend his remaining few days at home.

I arrived at their house without knowing what I was going to do. There I met a charming 9-year-old boy, Mickey, diagnosed with a malignant cancer and about to die. He sat there beside his grandmother, waiting for me, with her supporting his head—his brain was active, but he lacked the strength to keep his head upright. His mother was sitting near his grandmother, with Dan, Mickey's younger brother and witness to his sibling's slow and painful death. When Mickey's mother told me that his birthday was in two months, I immediately decided that we would celebrate it that very day. I announced to Mickey and the family that the festivities were beginning, starting with a performance by Madame Esther (my finger puppet) and followed by a magic show and then birthday songs and activities, including silly tasks to be performed by the family. Mickey was happy, laughing and enjoying himself. I thought to myself how happy I was to be with Mickey in that moment, and how amazing he was. I made a silent wish for him to live until Thursday so that I could come again and hear his laughter, and perhaps bring him a shell from Sponge Bob's beach to accompany him there.

After I said goodbye to Mickey and exited to the stairwell, his mother came up to me, and said that she had not heard him laugh like that for years, and thanked me.

But Mickey passed away before I could see him again. I called his mother to extend my condolences, and her chilling monologue—the eulogy of a mother—remained with me for a long time:

Mickey was such a good soul, what a life he had, with his short life—out of his nine years, he was battling his illness for the last three. He had no childhood. Nothing helped. With all of the treatments, the illness only became more aggressive. We couldn't do a thing. How can we go on now, how is it possible to go on? Mickey understood everything, children understand everything. On the day he died, he said, "Mommy, I'm going to die." That's how he said it. His last words were, "Mommy, Mommy." He always understood what was happening to him. He said to me, "Mom, don't cry." After we celebrated his birthday, he sat there, smiling. I teased him and asked him, "How come you're smiling now?" "Mom, I'm happy."—that's what he said. I don't know how I can go on now. When I go into his room, I hear him in my head, saying to me, "Good morning, Mom. How are you?" He was our firstborn. I hope that we have finished our portion of sorrow in life. It's difficult. I hope we won't experience any more sorrow. He had no pains. I was afraid he would go blind. At least that didn't happen. It's been so painful for his siblings. They were so close. His dad says that now it's easier for him "up there." Thanks for phoning.

Working with the terminally ill is a huge emotional challenge for the medical clown. The extent of the medical clown's involvement in his work is unique for each one—some hold back from too much emotional engagement while others don't. My condolence call to the late Mickey's mother was not part of my clown's job (or perhaps it was). The death of a child is especially saddening and enraging; for weeks after, I walked around with a feeling of deep distress and just could not stop thinking about Mickey. To give vent to some of that, I sat down to write. The result is the following strange sad–funny dialogue, throwing down the gauntlet:

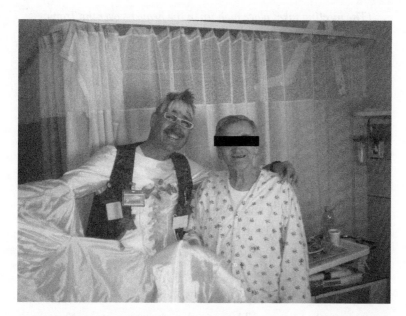

FIGURE 2.3 (ABOVE). A patient with the medical clown. Chaim Sheba Medical Center, Tel HaShomer, 2013.

FIGURE 2.4 (BELOW). Medical clown sings with a patient. Chaim Sheba Medical Center, Tel HaShomer, 2013.

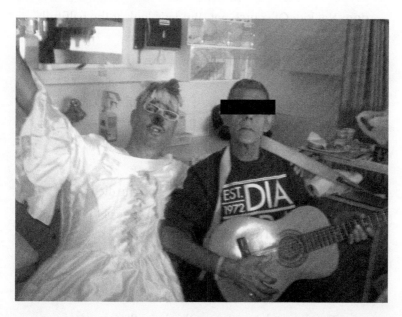

(*The meeting takes place high up in the heavens over the Tropic of Cancer*).

MICKEY. Where am I? Where's Mom and Dad?

GOD (*scratching the back of His neck uncomfortably*). Sorry, kid. Let me take you on a little walk through the Garden of Eden, I'll buy you something.

MICKEY. Who are you?

GOD (*pointing to a name tag on his lapel*). Elohim . . . God . . . Allah . . . I have a lot of names.

MICKEY. I have only one—Mickey. I was a boy, I got sick, and I died. I miss Dad and Mom and Grandma and . . .

GOD (*uneasy*). Ahmm . . . Sorry, kid. Don't make a big deal of this. You're not the only one.

MICKEY. Why?

GOD. Look, I have problems in the creation system. There are repetitive flaws and I haven't succeeded in solving them. It's hard for me to explain, and you're young.

MICKEY. Am I going to grow up?

GOD. No, kid. Of course not. But let's look at the half-full glass—at least you're not hurting here.

MICKEY. It hurts me about the life I didn't live, about Mom and Dad.

GOD (*leafing through His list in deep thought*). I can bring your mom here if you want.

MICKEY. No. That would be terrible for my brother.

GOD. Maybe a friend?

MICKEY. I had a friend in the hospice, but he died.

GOD. So he's here already. Ah . . . perhaps one of the clowns down there? There are some who are very old already, and there are always accidents, maybe a disease, we can arrange something.

MICKEY (*surprised*). Who?

GOD. There are a lot . . . let me think . . . there are lots . . .

MICKEY. Do you think they can make us laugh here, too?

GOD. Don't know. (*To Himself*) Down there they're not all that great . . . kinda pathetic. (*To Mickey*) I have no idea, they still haven't come up here. There was one who almost arrived two years ago . . . something with his heart . . . but at the end, it was cancelled.

MICKEY. Is there anyone here who knows how to hug? How to make us laugh?

GOD (*mulling*). The truth is there isn't. I'm busy with all of the faults and have no time for nonsense. And as for the angels, they're a bunch of morons I don't know what to do with.

MICKEY. OK, so maybe one of the clowns after all . . .

GOD. OK, kid, let me check it out. (*To Himself*) OMG! These bald kids know how to manipulate, guilt feelings, guilt feelings. (*Calls out to one of the angels.*) Daniel, see what you can do about those clowns.

It is important to note that the medical clown's performance for adults is entirely different from their performance for children, and their performance for patients with minor illnesses is totally different from their performance for patients with incurable diseases, or those who are dying slowly. What truly challenges the medical clown, both emotionally and professionally, is working with the terminally ill—they must marshall all of their emotions and their professional insights in order to create a performance that is most suitable for the patient.

Based on my experience with ill adults hospitalized in various departments, I can say that the adults are as much in need of a medical clown as the children. Therefore, a change in the approach to medical clowning in hospitals is needed so as to engage more and more medical clowns with adult and the elderly patients, especially those who are terminally ill. Medical clowning should be an option for every patient everywhere in the world.

CHAPTER THREE

The Healing Performance

The Medical Clown Compared with African !Kung and
Azande Ritual Healers

The medical clown, the drama therapist, the traditional healer, and
the witchdoctor each conduct a dramatic, theatrical healing performance with the objective of healing the ill in their community.
Their healing ability lies in their capacity to be intermediaries
between different worlds, between chaos and order, between the
factors which have caused or accelerated the illness and the healing
mental powers. Each healer, using his own unique practice embodied in the perception of reality in their community, facilitates access
to healing powers. This chapter will attempt a comparative study
of various healing performances in the context of their indigenous
culture and shared experiences.

Practice, Mediation, and Liminality

"The medical clown is a unique artist who performs in front of
patients and whose goal is to assist in the healing process of those
hospitalized in medical centers and convalescent homes" (Raviv
2012a: 170). Medical clowning has what Pendzik and Raviv called
"a family resemblance to drama therapy"(2011). Shamanism is
considered a precursor of both drama therapy and therapeutic
clowning; both share some characteristics in their methods and
practice, and use the same theatrical framework to help strengthen
and heal the patients. According to a 2011 study, medical clowning
differs from drama therapy for the patients perceive the clown as
an archetypal liminal figure and not as a therapist. In other words,
the drama therapist would be generally perceived by clients as

someone who belongs to ordinary reality, who may lead them or join them in a round trip into an imaginary world, but whose starting point is everyday reality. In contrast, "medical clowns, are generally perceived by their audience as belonging to the imaginary world. Throughout their interaction, the clown is seen not as a therapist but as a character from the imaginary realm" (ibid.: 273).

Linda Miller Van Blerkom presents one of the most interesting analyses of medical clowning by considering the medical clown as a modern shaman (1995). The medical context of the performance, the dramatic means, the language as well as the 'mediation' between the sources of power and strength is common among ritual healers (Handelman 1981). The objective of the performances by the medical clown, the !Kung healer, and the Azande witchdoctor are to heal or aid the healing process; they all use theatrical means and attire to intensify the dramatic effect as well as music (voice and instruments), audience participation, and dramatic role-playing. Illness introduces chaos into the world, bringing disorder into health and the natural order of individual and social life, and "both clowns and shamans mediate between order and chaos, sacred and profane, real and supernatural, culture and anti-culture, or nature" (Van Blerkom 1995:46).

The essence of the medical clown's mediation differs from the healer's, the shaman's, and the witchdoctor's, since the medical clown mediates between mental resources which already exist in every human being—humor and fantasy. Illness, pain, and anxiety tend to block this capacity, making it difficult for the patient to access the realms of humor and imagination; thus, the patient requires the medical clown's mediation to be 'transported' to those realms. Humor enables the patient to gaze at reality from a different perspective, from a more detached viewpoint, allowing the patient to experience reality without being intimidated by it.

The mediating practice of the healer and the witchdoctor differ from the medical clown in a fundamental aspect. Marjorie Shostak's (1981) ethnographic works describe an !kung healer who enters into a trance and arouses the healing power, or "*Num*," in order to leave his body to wander the world of spirits and meet the spirit or god with whom he must negotiate for the soul of the ill person. Shostak illustrates this with the story of a woman who fell ill after her father passed away. During the course of the ceremony, the healer "exited" his body to meet with the father's spirit which was holding tightly to his daughter's soul. The healer had to persuade the father's spirit, who wanted his daughter close to him, to let go of her since she had more to accomplish in the world of the living. The result was that the daughter recovered following the ritual in which the healer had mediated between the worlds on behalf of the audience, acting as an intermediary between the world in which they live and the mystical world of the spirits. The healer can access the world of the spirits unlike the audience, and thus bring about healing through the performance by engaging them in a deeply ritualistic discourse.

In contrast, the mediating practice of the witchdoctor of the Azande tribe is different. With the help of his trance and potion, the witchdoctor can "see" the witchcraft. As described by Evans-Pritchard, "An Azande witchdoctor is essentially a man who knows what plants and trees compose the medicines which, if eaten, will give him power to see witchcraft with his own eyes, to know where it resides, and to drive it away from its intended victims" (1976: 73). The witchdoctor's vision is two-sided: one, he can see what is hidden (what the spell is and who has cast it), not only regarding illness but also with a broader vision which encompasses varied issues such as crop cycles, family relationships, and more. These are capacities shared by shamans from other continents too, all over the world. Two: his ability to physically see the place where the spell has caused an injury to the body and caused or aggravated the illness. This is the exclusive ability of the witchdoctor which enables him to formulate a solution for the healing to take place.

In order for the medical clown, the healer, and the witchdoctor to be able to mediate between order and chaos, they must become liminal figures with the ability to pass through or bridge realities:

"It is a passage from ordinary reality, to that of ritual [. . .] predicated upon bypassing such anomalies of perception" (Handelman 1981: 322).

The !kung healer passes out of corporeal reality into the parallel reality of the world of spirits, seeking answers and solutions to the illness. The witchdoctor accomplishes passage and mediation through their ability to "see" spells as a form of protection and healing, to "see" the witchcraft in the body of the ill person and then distinguishing whether they have been harmed and fallen ill.

The medical clown's liminality is distinct from that of the healer or witchdoctor—while the !kung healer's and Azande witchdoctor's process takes place in front of their audience, the medical clown has already "arrived" from a "different" place to "sweep the audience away" into a world of humor and fantasy.

In comparison to the various healing performances, I will now present three vignettes from my work in various hospital wards over the years, which will illustrate the work of the medical clown.

The Biker

During my tenure at the oncology day unit in Chaim Sheba Medical Center, I met Ron, a patient, about 60 years old. He was seated in an armchair set up for patients, one among others in the room, all of them connected to their IV lines, preparing to receive chemotherapy which would take several hours. Since he visited the hospital quite a few times over the next few months, I was able to get to know him better. When I learned that he had been a biker, I devised a ritual for our encounters: I would mount an imaginary motorbike and make sounds of loudly gunning the motor at very high RPMs and "bike" around with Ron; I would "perform" daredevil acts, and he would join me, holding onto the virtual handlebar (while seated) and we would swerve around extremely dangerous mountain curves, driving down to the sea. As we rounded the curves on the "road," we would lean sideways, passing all of the other vehicles on the way. After our quick, uber-adventurous "ride,"

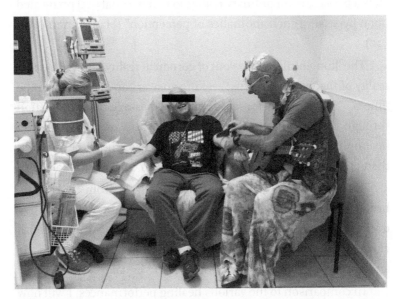

FIGURE 3.1 (ABOVE). The medical clown often assists the hospital staff during a medical procedure. Chaim Sheba Medical Center, Tel HaShomer, 2013.

FIGURE 3.2 (BELOW). The medical clown sings to a patient in the dialysis care unit. Harzfeld Hospital, Gedera, 2014.

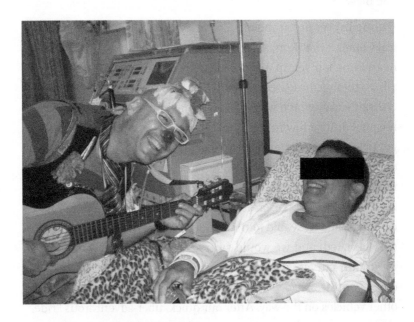

we would arrive at our destination, "dismount" with much laughter as we talked about the precarious trip.

Susana Pendzik points out the significant difference between the mediation and journey accomplished by the shaman in their healing performance and the process of the drama therapist. The shaman sets out alone on the journey, leaving his patients behind, mediating for them from a different place with superhuman forces. In contrast, the drama therapist, and like him, the medical clown, set out on a shared journey with their patients and mediate between them and the powers of imagination.

Ron, as a biker, "liberated" himself from his current reality through the power of imagination, and joined me on the journey. Two realities—one of the hospital, and the second of the imagination—coexist and the patient must choose the alternative one in response to his needs, when circumstances excruciatingly limit him. In our alternative reality, Ron and I were riding motorcycles. As Richard Schechner observes in *The Future of the Rituals* (1993), playacting is a creative act with a power that does not declare its true intention. The true intention of medical clowning is to take the patient, through play, on an imaginary journey in order to facilitate a healing dialogue with the grim reality in which he finds himself.

Magic Dust

Jack was a 6-year-old boy who had been hospitalized for several weeks at Chaim Sheba Medical Center due to severe pain in his bones. He spent most of his time in his wheelchair or in bed. His pain was intense, and often, when I visited, I found him in tears. So I had Madame Esther, my finger puppet, perform for him along with Shumi, the Green Frog. Then I conducted our special ritual: I would take some "magic dust" from the flower on my head, mix it with the magic dust from the flower on my lapel, then sprinkle it on the spots Jack pointed out as specially painful. I would whisper funny "spells," in gibberish, interspersed with statements about the pain disappearing immediately. To an adult observer, it might seem

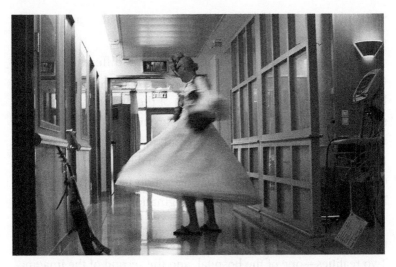

FIGURE 3.3 The medical clown at the Rabin Medical Center, Petach Tikva, 2015. *Photograph by Hezi Panet.*

as if the ritual were a parody, but for 6-year-old Jack the pains were truly lessened and often vanished completely.

It has been rightly noted through several years of research on cognitive responses that repetitive suggestions indeed lessen the pain. The patient's belief that the medical clown or shaman can heal or assist the healing through their performance does have an impact on their recovery. The placebo effect is the proof that human beings have inherent self-healing powers which may be activated by means of suggestion and association.

Jack, like the shaman's audience of ill persons, apparently believed that I had the capacity to lessen his pains by means of my magic dust; and this belief helped the maghic dust accomplish its aim. Adults, as well as children, believe that the medical clown's performance helps them feel better which in turn helps them overcome their illness and the disturbing reality of suffering.

One of my encounters with Jack was out of the ordinary. My daughter fell ill and had to be hospitalized in the same pediatric unit where I worked as a medical clown. That night, as I slept in her room by her side, I could hear Jack crying in the next room and

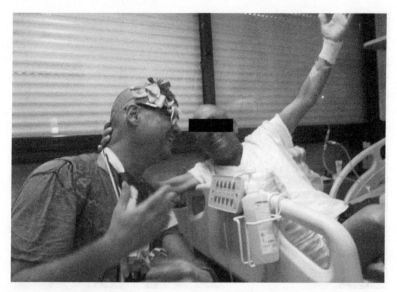

FIGURE 3.4 The medical clown's performance comprises theatrical aural–visual elements involving the patient who is not only the audience but also a co-performer. Chaim Sheba Medical Center, Tel HaShomer, 2013.

the soft voices of his parents who were unable to calm him. I went into his room and stood near his bed. I "gathered" magic dust out of the air, sprinkled it over his hurting body, then sang him a lullaby. Jack stopped crying, wiped his tears, and slowly drifted off to sleep. It seems he had no trouble maintaining my clown persona even when I was without my "bag of tricks."

Dance of the Eyebrows

I accompanied Mahmood since he was 6 months old and hospitalized at Chaim Sheba Medical Center for a genetic intestinal illness. In hospital, he was affected with a severe bacterial infection and had to be intubated and anesthetized in the ICU so that the doctors could strugle to save his life. He did survive, but the infection had been so severe that his hands and feet had to be amputated when he was 2 and half years old. Before the amputation, Mahmood loved to dance the wild dances with me, to the rhythm I drummed on the back of my guitar. After the surgery, when he

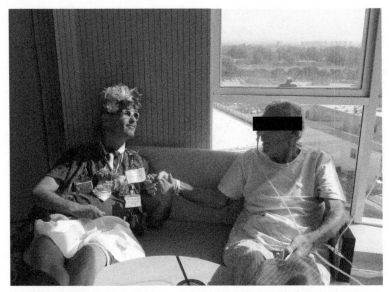

FIGURE 3.5 The medical clown creates a carnivalesque world within the hospital.
Chaim Sheba Medical Center, Tel HaShomer, 2016.

was no longer able to dance, we developed the "eyebrow dance,"
each of us wiggling our eyebrows to the beat my fingers tapped out
on the guitar.

Whenever Mahmood had to undergo a medical procedure,
almost all of which were very painful, even a blood test (because
the doctor had to take blood from a vein in his neck), I would stand
near him, and beating out a rapid rhythm on my guitar, do the eyebrow dance. Mahmood would laugh out loud, and was often able
to overcome his pain and ignore the needle. When the pain was
too much to bear, he would scream but then return to the eyebrow
dance and laughter. And so it would go on: between screams and
laughter. Mahmood cried during the procedures, but also laughed
during the dance of the eyebrows.

For the shaman and their audience as well as for the medical
clown and the patient, the dance and the beat lead to a unique state
of consciousness. Although the medical clown and the patient do
not enter a trance (as the shaman does), the medical clown, like

the stage actor, is in an altered state of consciousness yet is not entirely cut off from reality.

Mahmood also made the transition to an altered state of consciousness to dissociate himself from the pain, using the beat of my guitar-tapping and the "dance of the eyebrows". But when the pain intensified, he was drawn back into the normal state of consciousness. Shamanism is the most ancient method of linking body and soul for healing, and medical clowning is essentially shamanism adapted to the consensus of modern medicine. The medical clown's patients are assisted by rhythm and music to create a conscious state separated from the painful lived reality.

Handelman wrote extensively about the Ik tribe of northern Uganda who were forced to live on a reservation in dire poverty, near starvation, and in great despair. Laughter was their way to cope with hunger and pain. Each time several people gathered together, they began to laugh. This was their response and weapon against despair. Laughter is the human being's expression of opposition to his existential state (Bakhtin 1984; Fiske 1989a). Young Mahmood's laughter—the laughter of a little boy without hands or feet, with his burden of suffering—was his expression of opposition to his unbearable condition.

CHAPTER FOUR

The Clown's Carnival in the Hospital

A Semiotic Analysis of the Medical Clown's Performance

The medical clown's multimodal performance takes place within the rigid space of the hospital. That is to say, a clown in a hospital is a paradox. "Medical clowning" is a metaphor taken from two seemingly unrelated fields, juxtaposing the medical, the scientific, and the serious with the carnival spirit, emotions, and humor. The clown addresses barriers created by illness, pain, alienation, and distress with a continuous yet flexible performance of humor and fantasy, tailored to the specific conditions and circumstances of his audience. A clown, by definition, challenges the public order, and apprently has no place in a hospital. Within the purview of this argument we can attempt to compare medical clowns to carnival clowns, examine their performance, and present a semiotic analysis of the clown's journey through the hospital, assessing the significance of his performance on an ideological level.

On Carnivals and Clowning

The roots of the carnival lie deep in ancient rituals, such as the Dionysia in ancient Greece and the Saturnalia in ancient Rome. In *Rabelais and His World* (1984), Bakhtin argued that the carnival culture had great significance during the Middle Ages and the Renaissance. Mocking the official "truth" and the power of the Church, and constituting an opposition or, rather, an alternative to the regime, carnival laughter "built its own world in opposition to the official world" (Bakhtin 1984: 88) and is characterized by "its indissoluble and essential relation to freedom" (ibid.: 89).

Carnival laughter had healing qualities, and carnival masks were associated with joy, reincarnation, and transformative change. In medieval culture, carnival laughter was also able to transform the frightening into the funny, thus lessening or nullifying the level of threat embodied by the frightful. The medical clown makes use of this characteristic in his attempt to lessen patients' anxiety in hospitals.

Bakhtin reasoned that medieval man lived in two worlds, the official world and the carnival world. The serious and carnival coexisting as separate entities, and this duality and transition between the two worlds created the balance in life. The carnival played a significant role in liberating the individual from subjectivity and ideology, as it presented the body and accessibility to the body in and of itself; the body at carnival time did not signify something else but referred only to its own drives and denotative-material presence. Carnival celebrated life in its basic, existential, physical-bodily essence, as a liberation of the individual from hierarchical, ideological, and social consensus. Moreover, it suspended the social order and hierarchy and invented, in direct opposition to the norm, its own modus operandi. Carnival crowned the clown as the king of misrule, a king who nullified and mocked all social orders and ideologies.

Bakhtin describes carnival as characterized by laughter, exaggeration, bad taste, insults; it turns things upside down and brings forth a sense of equanimity. Carnival involves a connection to the primordial, irrepressible powers which are alien to any idea of social control. Because of this, carnival and other carnivalesque events bear a potential threat to the social order, which is compelled to enforce moral and aesthetic laws to rein in the threat. All regimes are threatened by carnival, because it is a reminder of the fragility of social control. Bakhtin described the phenomenon of the fairs. Widespread in medieval Europe, the fairs comprised popular entertainments by clowns and fools, together with bizarre performances before a drunken, riotous crowd loudly celebrating their opposition to the prevailing social order. Such was the disorder that King Henry VI enacted limiting orders and established the Court of Piepowders for the period of the fairs as the exclusive agency empowered to handle the riots that inevitably broke out during this time.

In modern times, the fair was displaced to locations set up on the outskirts of towns, and its time was taken over by the official national holiday whose significance derived from the world of labor. "Holiday" belongs to the world of manufacturing, subject to the ideology of the consumer society, while carnival celebrates the body and expresses opposition to ideology. The goal of official holidays from work is to provide the laborer with a short vacation all the better to return to work and be even more productive. John Fiske stated that ideology in Western (capitalist consumer) societies owe their power and validity to their being perceived as natural and logical by all members of society, even the enslaved (1990). Basing his arguments on Marxist thought, and the work of theorists such as Louis Althusser and Antonio Gramsci, he surmised that ideology has the capacity to contain, refine, and integrate the carnivalesque and expressions of protest into the social systems it creates. Clowning is one excellent example of this capacity.

The clown was one of the dominant carnivalesque figures in human history: "The clown was first disguised as a king. But once his reign had come to an end, his costume was changed ('travestied') to turn him once more into a clown"(Bakhtin 1984: 197). The clown is the ultimate carnival figure and diametrically opposite to the king. As figures of protest against order and discipline, expressing the oppression of the masses, clowns were taken off the streets in the name of social order and transferred to restricted areas enabling supervision and control. The carnival clown was refined and recruited to the service of society, and thus turned into just another entertainer at "cultural festivals." An excellent illustration of the refining the carnival clown (and the circus clown) may be seen in Tod Browning's film *Freaks* (1932), which takes place in a traveling-circus sideshow. Browning filmed authentic midgets and clowns with deformities who were an integral part of a circus. The response to the film was extremely critical and it was heavily censored because viewers could not bear to see the physical deformities. While Fiske noted that deformity is the opposite of the Western ideal of beauty, the deformed clown's body presents an insufferable challenge to the aesthetics of perfection which represent and "reflect" the integrity of society.

The Medical Clown

The literature on medical clowning refers to the carnivalesque with regard to three aspects of the work of the medical clown. The first refers to the laughter the clown arouses to reduce anxiety among hospitalized patients. Hansen and his colleagues in 2011 reported on children's laughter elicited by medical clowns' antics (during botulinum toxin injections) which helped reduce the child–patients' anxiety. Previous studies have also suggested that laughter lessened anxiety among children when a medical clown accompanied them or performed for them in the operating room, especially, before surgeries. In my various articles, I have described the medical clowns' practice of treating trauma victims in hospitals, both children and adults in shock from artillery fire and rockets landing near their homes or schools. Arriving at the emergency room, they received "first aid" from the medical clowns—grotesque humor and carnivalesque laughter. The outcome was a drastic drop in their anxiety. This was further evinced in the report by Dafna Tener and colleagues in 2010, which documented the success of a female medical clown's performance among girls who were victims of sexual abuse.

The second aspect refers to the healing power of carnival laughter. As Van Blerkoom states, the medical clown is "the modern shaman" with the ability to heal through carnivalesque laughter. The liminal performance by the clown and shaman mediates between chaos and order, between the wild and the domesticated or civilized. In an article published in 2011, Pendzik and I analyzed several case studies in order to derive that the laughter and imagination the medical clown arouses in patients is therapeutic. An additional study that was conducted over one year in a hospital by Prof. Shevach Friedler among 219 in-vitro fertilization patients found that the appearance of a medical clown during treatment improved their success rates of becoming pregnant compared to the group which was not exposed to a medical clown's performance.

The third aspect is the carnivalesque opposition to repression. Both Citron and I have argued that the medical center is a hierarchical and rigid structure in which patients lose part of their identity and independence—they patients must wear "uniforms", are often tied to their beds with an IV line, and always subject to the medical staff's authority. The medical clown's carnivalesque laughter arouses the patients' opposition to this alienated state along with the depression often brought on by the illness. The very fact that they are rebelling against their dislocated and weakened states strengthens their souls and enlivens their mood.

The medical clown is a new breed of clown, recruited to the service of the society. He brings the carnival to a place that seems least suitable—to the hospital, to where life encounters death. According to Bakhtin, "In the act of carnival laughter, death and resurrection mix . . . This is the world-embracing laughter, so very universal. This is its unique special quality, the specification of ambivalent laughter" (1978: 130). The carnivalesque opposes not only the social order but also the cosmic, protesting the fragile existence of humans in the face of Death. This is the spirit of carnival laughter, the celebration of life itself, that very same untrammelled, untamed energy bursting out uncontrollably, mocking illness and death. It is the binary opposite of fear, and a powerful weapon in the human arsenal to overcome the fear of death. It is the affirmation of life. As Allen Klein states, "With each laugh the clown elicits from us, he reminds us that out of death can come an affirmation of life" (1998: 51).

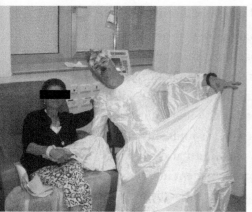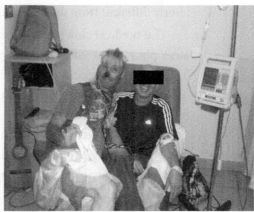

FIGURE 4.1 and **4.2** (LEFT, RIGHT). The clown's performance must be customized for the patient in keeping with their needs in the most personal and precise manner. The medical clown assists two patients undergoing treatment at Chaim Sheba Medical Center, Tel HaShomer, 2015.

The narrative of the medical clown in the Western healthcare delivery system is relatively new. It describes the medical clown as assisting the healing process of patients through humor and fantasy, and rests upon studies which point to humor and laughter being good for one's health because modern medicine needs an official "stamp of approval" in order to allow the clown's entrance into and acceptance by the hospital paradigm. In fact, the medical establishment's acceptance of the hypothesis that laughter is the best medicine paved the way for the medical clown's entrance into the rigid hospital hierarchy.

The biopic *Patch Adams* (1998) on the "father of medical clowning" depicts the story of Dr. Hunter Dohery "Patch" Adams's years as a medical student, and quickly became an essential part of the myth of the medical clown. In *Television Culture* (1992), Fiske argued that fashion in clothing is one of the expressions of the carnivalesque in films; indeed, in the film, the more determined Patch Adams becomes to oppose the medical establishment, the more his style shifts from conservative to flamboyant and ornate. The medical clown stands out with his wild, extraordinary sartorial style, so utterly different from the staff and patient uniforms.

The medical clown is a liminal figure who arrives from "another place" in a built-in real-life paradox. He belongs, yet does not belong, to the medical staff, creating what Jean Baudrillard in *Simulacra and Simulation* (1994) has called dissimulation—disguising reality, and simulation, creating a fantasy-like reality within the space of the hospital. At times, the clown's liminality is expressed in not belonging to the hospital paradigm; at other times, it is expressed in his ability to transport the patient into the realms of humor and imagination. As in all carnivals, the audience is an active participant in the performance, even in the hospital.

The clown's dominant denotative sign is the red nose, a bit of plastic or other material, sometimes simply red paint. The red nose signifies the carnival spirit and drunkenness (since a red nose is characteristic of drunkards). The red nose, in the spirit of carnival,

FIGURE 4.3 This carnival performance is what the medical clown brings into the specific site of the medical facility which is why the clown is, to a certain extent, a site-specific artist. Rabin Medical Center, Petach Tikva, 2015. *Photograph by Hezi Panet.*

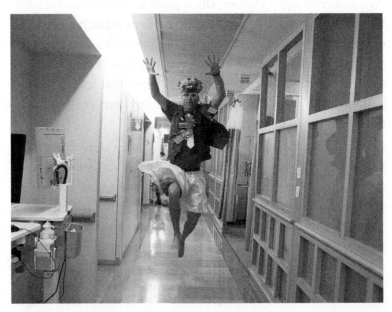

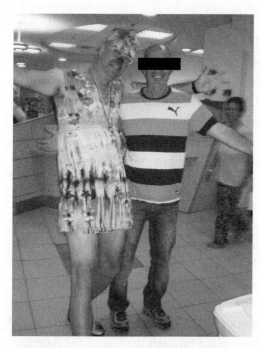

FIGURE 4.4 A family member of a patient with the medical clown at Chaim Sheba Medical Center, Tel HaShomer, 2015.

challenges the hierarchical structure and creates emotional whirlpools between patients and staff, and between patients and patients, yet it is precisely because of this that it empowers the patient in both spaces: the first space is external to the patient, that is, the space of the staff, the medical procedures, the interaction with other patients and the overwhelming hospital building. Coping with such a loss of territory, and of identity, would be difficult even for a healthy person. The second space is the internal space where the patient must cope with emotions and other difficulties arising from the illness.

The First Case Study

M is a Kurdish child from Iraq, hospitalized in the intensive cardiac care unit at Chaim Sheba Medical Center, seated in a wheelchair with his mother by his side. That's how I met him as I entered the room. I immediately took out my Arabic–Hebrew medical dictionary and proceeded to question M, in minute detail, about his farts and his bowel movements. His initial confusion very quickly turned into laughter as I demonstrated, with the help of a "fart generator" hidden in my back pocket, the correct way to fart. Then I began to drum on the back of my guitar, as if it were a darbouka, to the rhythm of the "farts" and M began to move about in his wheelchair and make fart sounds with his mouth. When the nurse came in to check what the noise was all about in her otherwise quiet department, she couldnn't help but join in our game.

The analysis of the case begins with the fact that it involved a Kurdish child hospitalized in a foreign country, far away from home. Dislocated and displaced into a grim white room. The clown's sense of non-belonging to the medical staff or the hospital locale and culture enabled the child to bond with him. "The clown is always an outsider, acting from the border, blurring hierarchies and challenging authority. This ability to operate from the margins allows them to help where others fail" (Pendzik and Raviv 2011: 272). The initial connection took place through the use of the Arabic–Hebrew medical dictionary to ask routine questions which then became grotesque and crude. The earthiness of the farts and the noisy celebratory atmosphere express the carnivalesque opposition to the sterility of the hospital and the child's feeling of loss of control. The clown also helps break down the child's invisible barrier with the nurse who was only too happy for an opportunity to participate in the festivities.

The Second Case

Y is a man about 60 years old, whom I have known for a long time, since he is a dialysis patient at Hartzfeld Geriatric Hospital. About a week before my visit, he underwent a second leg amputation, followed by a cardiac incident. Patients in the dialysis department sit near the dialysis machines that are so huge that you cannot see past them. The TV screens mounted in the center of the room emit a bothersome, monotonous buzz. The nurses sit at their station, and walk through the patients from time to time, monitoring and noting their blood pressure or recording data from the machines. When I stood near Y that morning, tears began to run down his face. "I'm sick of this. I'm giving up. I want it to be over." I looked into his teary eyes for several seconds, and putting my left hand on his right, I approached him as if I were going to tell him a great secret. "'Listen,' I said, "it's great that they took off the second leg. You've already got used to doing everything 'on one foot.' Besides, now you can ask for medical marijuana. So go ahead, order a large amount, and we'll party here in the ward." I turned to B, another double amputee sitting beside Y, "We're having a dance party, Y is bringing the 'grass'. Can you arrange the lights and music?" "Sure, I also have tap dancing shoes," he said. Then I began dancing to trance music in front of Y, making drum movements and sounds and Y, staring at me, slowly began to smile through his tears.

In this case, we had an elderly dialysis patient exhibiting acute distress. It is important to note that the medical clown and the patient had a long-term acquaintance, and the patient relayed a muted call for help across a room full of people. The call and the connection was acknowledged through their gazes, with the added physical touch of hands, to convey the message "I am here for you" as well as "I am taking you with me into the realm of the unreal." Black humor also engages the other patient, especially the idea of a grotesque dance. This further elucidates that the alternative point of view facilitates a distant, absurdly humorous perspective for the patient and effectively alleviates pain and anxiety. In C. E. Carp's words: "The clown with its archetypal power, multicultural history, crazy wisdom, hilarious antics and paradoxical nature is the quintessential character to guide the individual on a healing journey" (1998: 254).

The Third Case

B passed away at the ripe old age of 85. When I arrived at Hartzfeld Hospital, her lifeless body lay in bed, surrounded by her mourning family. I had gotten to know her during the last month of her life, and used to sing her old French and Italian songs while dancing with an invisible partner. She would smile, seated at her little table, strapped securely into her wheelchair. When I stopped into her room for a visit three days before she died, I found her stretched out in bed, drained of strength, her eyes closed. I leaned closer and began to sing a song, composed on the spot, with simple words from all the languages I knew: "B, I love you," and strummed my guitar, miming the face of a desperate suitor. B opened her eyes for a moment and looked at me, and a big smile spread over her fac. She made a tiny gesture as if to say, "You incurable romantic," then shut her eyes again, but the smile remained.

This is an example of a minimal yet effective performance—aquiet song sung into the ear of an elderly woman, the expression of a doomed lover, and nothing more. A longer interaction was beyond her strength. Her bright eyes, big smile, and small gesture of dismissal indicated the moment shared by B and the clown.

The healing performance by the medical clown is tailored for the patient. Which is why it is difficult to characterize it. At times it is an interaction in which the medical clown dances with the patient in the hospital room, accompanied by calls of encouragement and laughter from the other patients and their families. The stage is the hospital room. At other times, the performance may consist of a song sung quietly into the ear of the patient who is too weak to even sit up. In this situation, the "stage" is miniature, no more than the space between the performer's mouth and the patient's ear.

Sometimes the medical clown has no active partner for a performance, for the patient seems to ignore the clown's presence. However, ignorance does not necessarily mean that the patient wants the medical clown to go away.

A child was being treated in the burn unit. Screaming in pain he "did not notice the clown." But the next day he told his parents about the clown's visit, describing to the tiniest detail the clown's actions. In fact, it was only the clown's performance that the child retained from the otherwise painful day of treatment.

Sometimes the medical clown's performance includes the medical-care staff (their cooperation depends, of course, on their willingness to take part in the interaction with the medical clown and the patient). When the entire medical team participates in the interaction, it empowers the patient and brings a carnivalesque element into the hospital—it enables a reversal of the hierarchy: the patient, on the lowest rung, subject to medical authority and its binding recommendations, can now take command (assisted by the medical clown, of course). In the process, it creates an environment of camaraderie and trust. Besides the skills and capacities of the medical clown to create a carnivalesque world within the hospital space, they need to have a high degree of E.I.—emotional intelligence—in order to identify the right path to empower a particular patient, whether to reflect the patient's emotions through clownish actions and language or to express empathy or a share their own vulnerability.

Medical clowns do not create an alternative carnival world opposed to the serious world, but create a synthesis between the two. They are not operating in a "total world" but are committed to being extremely considerate of the consensus of the hospital. The hospital is a serious, hierarchical institution. Foucault drew parallels between the Middle Ages while calling modern physicians the "priests of the body." Within the synthesis that the medical clowns create in hospital, the medical staff is also committed to adopt, or at least to allow, the existence of the carnival laughter that the medical clown introduces for the patient's well-being.

Toward the end of *Patch Adams*, Robin Williams as Adams stands before a disciplinary panel of physicians who must decide whether to allow him to complete his medical studies. The head of the medical school accuses him of "excessive happiness" and humor which has no place in medicine. The panel decides that

Adams's humorous technique is not to their taste but find nothing wrong with it and allow him to complete his studies.

Now, 40 years after Adams's story, medical clowns are still met with opposition in medical centers. As today's medical clowns carve their way through adult wards (at present, clowning in pediatrics wards is common), they encounter raised eyebrows, lack of cooperation, and even concrete resistance from some of the medical staff. However, I must say that just as many medical staff are very pleased with their presence in the wards. Patients in the adult wards long for comic relief, and are in dire need of the medical clown's carnivalesque interventions, a celebration of life which links those who are ill to the primeval power of life, the life force which enables patients to combat their illness, fear, and alienation. The medical clown's performance is a healing performance linked to performances by the clown of the carnival and the shaman, touching upon the most intimate places in their audience, often at the critical juncture between life and death.

CHAPTER FIVE

On a Training and Evaluation Model for Medical Clowns

A set of guidelines ascertaining the standards is necessary to regularize medical clowning and to ensure its recognition as a paramedical practice in medical facilities across the world. Although duality and ambiguity are part of the medical clown's performance, there are six basic elements that are essential to the practice. And this chapter provides the necessary recommendations for the professional training and evaluation of medical clowns, especially those employed in a medical center.

I consider myself fortunate to have been working over the past decade as a partner helping shape medical clowning as a therapeutic discipline, and I am privileged to be teaching the subject at the university level. Since 2006, I have been an instructor in a pioneering course at University of Haifa, the first and possibly the only academic program in the world to grant a BA in Medical Clowning. Based on my teaching experience and my work as an active member of the Dream Doctors Project, I saw the need to set out an orderly description of a training and evaluation model.

The "Youngest Member" of the Family of Expressive Therapies
Medical clowning is the "baby" in the family of creative arts therapy, since only in recent years has it been consolidating its experience and rationale into a formal framework.

In 2011, Pendzik and I described the "family resemblance" between the medial clown and the drama therapist, emphasizing the essential nature of the work and the way in which both create an imaginary world, dramatic reality, and aesthetic distance. The most outstanding difference between the two, however, is that throughout the interaction with the patient, the clown is perceived as a performing artist—not a healer or caregiver. This is why it becomes an "invisible" encounter, an effective therapeutic process although not a conscious one (from the aspect of the patient). It is a creative, destabilizing action that frequently does not declare its existence, even less its intentions (Schechner 1983). The clown is able to interact with the patient directly and stimulate a therapeutic process that is entirely different from other types of creative arts therapies. The medical clown is not perceived as a creative arts performer or a therapist per se. Instead, an anomalous, liminal figure, the clown represents a realm of fantasy and humor whose performances are often impromptu and, therefore, not loaded with information or excessive content that prove difficult for patients, especially children. The anxiety related to encounters with authority (the establishment in general, and the healthcare system in particular) and the discomfort associated with negative self-image due to the need for care is eased in this manner.

In the 2010 article, "Laughing through This Pain," the researchers examined the function of the medical clown during examinations of child patients at the sexual assault victims treatment unit in Poriya Medical Center, and observed that the clowns could easily bond with the children and form an alliance against regimen, authority, officials, and the world of adults in general. The medical clown deftly responds to the need for peer-group identification and the need to rebel against authority that controls their lives.

A carnival performance is what the medical clown brings into the site of the medical facility, which is why the clown is, to a certain extent, a site-specific artist. From the aspect of the audience and the space, it may even be called a site-specific performance art. Miwon Kwon has described site-specific art as a form of surrender to the environmental context, since it is formulated or staged in the shadow of a specific site, as amalgamation or disruption, or a contrast with the site. This is an apt description of the work of the medical clown, which by its very nature cannot exist without the site (the professional medical space), and the "audience" which populates the site.

The medical clown's work is not a disruption or a contrast to the hospital but a catalyst that transforms the site. In a dualistic manner, the hospital becomes an "other" place of fantasy shared by clown and patient. International artists Christo and Jeanne-Claude's work concretizes the issues of the transformation of a locale. For example, their installation, *Wrapped Reichstag* (1995), which entailed wrapping the Reichstag building with silvery-white cloth to create "an 'other' place"—a fairy-tale castle. The medical clown also creates "an 'other' place" for the patient through a fantasy enacted with or without props.

Nick Kaye has described site-specific performance art as an examination of relationships and borders and the constant changes taking place on the borderlines between performer, site, and audience (2000). These are open relations in terms of flow, borders, stances, and changes. This description also fits the work of the medical clown, since the work is open, enables a flowing dialogue which changes according to audiences and sites, and constantly tests limits. The site-specific artist selects the site based on inspiration and free choice, which results in the art experience, while the clown doctor's choice is dictated by medical necessity. In the case of hospitalized patients, the link to the site is physical, for example, an IV line or bed rest, and the need to have an official release letter before leaving the premises. Both the actor and acted-upon in the clown–audience–site relationship are born out of medical necessity rather than aesthetic experience.

The fundamental difference between the interaction of the site-specific artist and his audience or the circus clown and his audience, and between the medical clown and his audience lies in the goal, mode of work, and selection of the site. While the performance artist or circus clown (or any other clown) strives to create an aesthetic experience or entertainment value, the goal of the medical clown is to assist in the healing process and, at times, to aid the family members of the patient to deal with difficulties and stress caused by the illness, and to promote better communication between them and healthcare professionals at the facility.

The Six Elements for Training and Evaluation of the Medical Clown

From the very first lesson, students specializing in medical clowning embark on an internal journey to discover their "inner" clown. This amusing and difficult journey takes a long time, and holds up a mirror to help the person reflect and understand the different aspects of their own personality. It often changes the way the students look upon life. This journey does not end with the course, nor upon graduation, but marks the beginning of a lifelong learning. The journey continues through their work over the years, as medical clowns in pediatrics, with PTSD patients, in oncology wards, with adult dialysis patients and in hospices for terminal patients. This is a journey that provides insights to those working in the field while constantly readjusting the lenses through which they look at life.

Students are not supposed to imitate any clown they may have seen, no matter how successful, nor should they create their clown by patching together aspects from here and there. They must work though it progressively; there is no archetype or role model in the field of medical clowning. Each clown should be different and unique to themselves.

The first element in discovering one's inner clown is the authentic and free connection to pleasure and joie de vivre. The second is the authentic connection to empathy and basic curiosity.

The work of the medical clown is the *clown interaction* between the clown and the patient (there are exceptions, such as singing to unconscious patients). In other words, medical clowning takes place when there is an interaction between the medical clown and the hospitalized patient based on clowning language (humor and fantasy) and tools (improvisations and gigs). This *interaction* can take

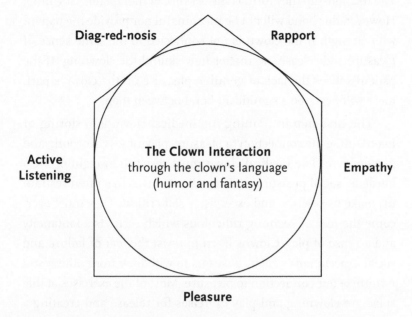

Diag-red-nosis   Rapport

Active
Listening

The Clown Interaction
through the clown's language
(humor and fantasy)

Empathy

Pleasure

FIGURE 5.1. The Six-Elements Model for training and evaluating the medical clown.

place optimally only when the other five elements support it: *pleasure, empathy, active listening, diag-red-nosis* (the diagnosis obtained from the clown's red nose), and *rapport.* Any flaw in any of the supportive "beams" damage the interaction (to a greater or lesser degree) between the medical clown and their patient/audience.

The training and evaluation of the medical clown must take place using these parameters: the quality of the interaction using clowning language expressed through the six elements. I will now focus on each of these elements and try to explain their nuances with a few practical examples.

Pleasure

The clown's connection to joie de vivre and pleasure powers the "generator" for the interaction with the patient. Unlike the circus clown who performs for a large audience, the medical clown works on a more one-to-one basis with an individual or a small group.

The relationship they form is the essence of therapeutic clowning. However, this bond will not be meaningful nor provide the patient with strength if the clown is not connected to the same sense of pleasure and release, no matter how skillful the clowning. If the patient senses the lack of genuine pleasure on the clown's part, there will never be a significant bond between them.

The first step in training the medical clown is restoring or maintaining the connection to pleasure, playfulness, freedom, and joie de vivre. The medical clown must resist the weight of life's burdens, social pressure, and social consensus that often restrain us, make us solemn, and excessively self-critical. They must overcome the fear of seeming ridiculous which restricts spontaneity and a sense of play. Clowns learn to resist the fear of failure and social expectations which causes us to withdraw from others and minimize our connection to pleasure. Most of the exercises at this stage are clowning and play exercises for release and creating a supportive atmosphere free of any self-criticism or group criticism which enables the candidates/students to feel secure enough to be free, ridiculous, and playful, and to be what is called in theater in the "here and now," in pleasure without the critical gaze.

The pleasure connection is not confined to the training period but is a constant accompaniment to the medical clown. Routine is the enemy of pleasure—the clowns must renew themselves and be renewed in order to "recharge their batteries." But pleasure's enemy is mental distress caused by witnessing difficult cases: painful suffering, death (in some cases, after years of battling an illness and years of friendship between the patient and the clown). At times, "renewal" is not enough to recharge, the clown may also need therapy (therapist as client—the healer in need of healing) in order to vent their feelings and avoid burnout. Many medical clowns, after years of working in the profession, report periods of fatigue, lack of desire, and a lessening of pleasure caused by emotional strain. Some may even quit. As Daniel Russell states, "Pleasure is actually an important part of how we live . . . pleasure

helps us do things and do them well" (2005: 1). This is true especially for the medical clown since creating and establishing mutual
pleasure with the patients is a critical component of their work.

Empathy

Robert L. Katz has written about the importance of empathy in any
healer–client relationship (1963). People sometimes ask why
patients need clowns at all; they can just watch comedies on the
TVs in their rooms. To them my answer is: patients need medical
clowns because the fundamental nature of the shared bond of
humor and fantasy, based on empathy, is enlivening. The clown is
the only one who transmits a personal message to the patient: I
"see" you, and I'm there for you, unlike the rest of the often largely
interpersonal medical staff and their attitude towards the patients.

Traditional medical training inculcates skills for diagnosis and
treatment but seems to neglect training and development in interpersonal skills. Although qualitative attributes such as interpersonal and communication skills, professionalism and the ability
to display and provide compassionate care are less tactile than
the skills used to diagnose and treat, they are equally vital to healing
patients.

Paul McGhee, after numerous studies, came up with a brilliant
distinction about the therapeutic nature of humor, especially with
regard to mental and physical health. According to him, having a
well-developed sense of humor is not enough to obtain the mental
health and resilience-boosting benefits, since a well-developed
negative sense of humor can end up interfering with good psychological health and effective social interaction (2010). This distinction is important and should be emphasized because humor is
usually perceived as a positive quality. But there are two types of
humor: positive humor which reinforces and empowers and connects people (and whose motive is empathy); and negative humor
humiliates, which mocks and divides people (and whose motive is
aggressiveness and dominance).

This is why it is so important to emphasize the role of empathy in a medical clown's interaction with the patient. The ability to empathize is associated with personality structure, education, and emotional intelligence and can be intensified through practice exercises.

Active Listening

Active listening is vital in order to map the emotional state of the patient and the patient's family, to understand the situation in the hospital room, and to gather information about what one is witnessing.

Active listening is the sine qua non of creating rapport and good interaction between the medical clown and the patient. There are various and simultaneous levels of listening which encompass much more than hearing, and which involve a combination of processes, including attention, hearing, understanding, and remembering. The concept of active listening refers to the assimilation of data through *all* ones senses. It is an in-depth contemplation of the people and their situation in order to understanding both better. The difference between receiving an oral message and actively listening is similar to the difference between scanning a textbook and reading it for comprehension and retention.

Larry L. Barker noted that the ego tends to reduce listening; in other words, the more the clown represses or neutralizes his ego, the higher the quality of his listening (1971). The training works to take one's ego out of the equation and encourages the students to develop their abilities at making themselves ridiculous and improving their active listening skills. Medical clowns must constantly remain in their active-listening mode, especially upon entering a hospital room. Active listening is what constantly directs the clown's activities throughout the time of their interaction with the patient.

Diag-red-nosis

The information received through active listening and an analysis of the patient and the patient's condition comprises the data processed by the medical clown into a "diag-red-nosis". The most important parameters under consideration for this are the patient's age, physical state and energy levels, mood and nature of interactions with family, friends, other patients and their environment, details about their hobbies and interests, and the type of visitors.

This information often comes from the patient or those around the patient and from items around their hospital bed, such as books, games, clothing, and so on. It is important to emphasize that the medical clown's active listening and diagnosis is *not* a stage necessarily followed by the interaction but, rather, is an extremely important process that takes place constantly through the interaction. The goal of the medical clown's active listening and "diag-red-nosis" is to facilitate a connection, based on rapport (sharing), and then to arrive at an interaction with the patient and those around the patient. That vital rapport cannot be developed without active listening and diag-red-nosis.

Rapport

The Oxford English Dictionary defines "rapport" as "a friendly relationship in which people understand each other very well" and provides an example that is relevant to the issue under discussion: *honesty is essential if there is to be good rapport between patient and therapist.*

Rapport is the good relationship that the medical clown builds with the patient, an empathic and genuine bond between individuals. A good rapport ensures that the patient is at ease with the medical clown, and shares an authentic, personal, and unique relationship with him. This bond in turn becomes the source of strength for the patient. However, rapport can be established only when all of the other elements are in place—that is, when there is genuine pleasure in the relationship between medical clown and patient.

In *The Healing Power of Humor* (1989), Klein refers to the importance of rapport in the context of laughter. To encourage laughing *with* people, not at them, we need to establish a rapport with the people. It is an error to perceive that the essential work of the medical clown is to make his audience laugh. Rather, it is the relationship he builds with his patients/audience, based upon a sensitively and empathetically developed rapport.

The Clown Interaction

The medical clown's interaction with the patient rests, of course, on all of these elements, on the clowning language and tools organized within the framework of creative improvisations and gags. The medical clown uses all of the classical forms of humor (incongruity, opposites, exaggeration, minimization, the absurd), but the humor that the medical clown shares with the patient has much broader ramifications than its classical components. The function and the significance of humor for the patient are greater than among the healthy, or those who are merely seeking entertainment.

Klein in *The Courage to Laugh* (1998), discussing the significance of humor and its use among the ill, uses"humor" in its broadest sense, as a metaphor for a full range of positive emotions: hope, joy, pleasure, fun, happiness, celebration, optimism, and the will to live. And McGhee describes humor as hope among cancer patients; many cancer patients have said that being able to laugh through their treatment helped sustain the sense of hope, that they could ultimately beat the disease (2010). Citing the many research studies on the importance of humor as a significant factor in the fight against cancer, he claims that several studies have demonstrated that humor *does* boost the activity of natural killer cells (which seek out and destroy malignant tumor cells). However, the most remarkable study he mentions was conducted in Norway over a seven-year period, in which the correlation between humor and

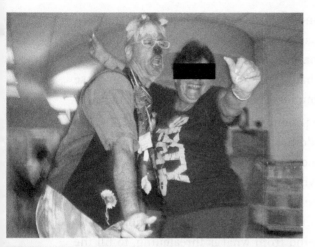

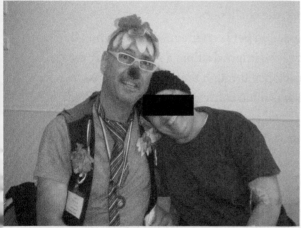

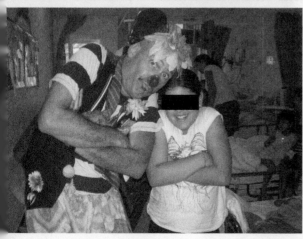

FIGURE 5.2 (TOP). With a family member of a patient at Chaim Sheba Medical Center, Tel HaShomer, 2013.

FIGURE 5.3 (MIDDLE). A good rapport ensures that the patient is able to feel at ease with the medical clown, and that they share an authentic, personal, and unique relationship. The medical clown with a patient at Chaim Sheba Medical Center, Tel HaShomer, 2010.

FIGURE 5.4 (BOTTOM). With a child patient at Barzilai Medical Center, Ashkelon, 2010.

recovery was studied among dozens of cancer patients. Immediately following diagnosis, a test was administered to the patients for their sense of humor. Those scoring higher on the test at the beginning of the study had a 70% higher survival rate than those with a poorer sense of humor. The results were unambiguous.

Humor enables the patient (of all ages) to hold on to life with a stronger grasp. In addition to the hope, humor enables the patient to remove some of the menace from their own condition. The fantasy that the clown creates enables the patient to experience "an 'other' place," as the fantasy alleviates the anxiety and stress related to complicated medical procedures. Imagination has the power to distract the mind from what is threatening, to fill the patient with strength to face the challenges.

The nature of the interaction between the medical clown and patient is a free-flowing creative improvisation, a spontaneous yet unexpected connection developed through the clowning language of humor and fantasy which is often conveyed through the gags (a gag can be anything that contains the element of "I have it in my bag of tricks", such as a joke, a magic trick, a finger puppet, a song, and so on).

Practical Training Exercises for the Medical Clown

Training and practice enables the clown to construct a persona, a language, and a toolbox while fine-tuning work on the basics of medical clowning. To obtain an initial idea of medical clowning, I shall present several examples of the type of exercises recommended for the training process. Of course, there are several exercises and different variations, and it is always possible to invent an infinite number of new drills.

A. SOME WARM-UP EXERCISES TO PRACTICE THE BASICS

1. *Dancing.* A group of at least three or more stand in a circle and dance to changing music. One of them begins and the others imitate his movements. The "leader" changes until

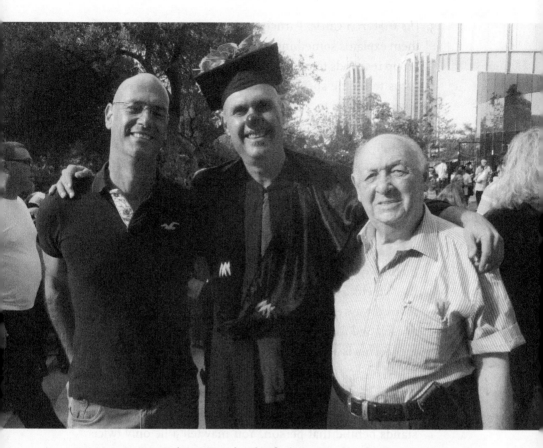

FIGURE 5.5 Amnon Raviv has received a PhD for his research on medical clowning for patients with life-threatening and incurable diseases. At the convocation ceremony with his father and brother. Haifa University, 2016.

everyone in the circle has had a chance to lead the dancing. **This is an exercise in enjoyment as a group, active listening, improvisation in movement, and coordination.**

2. *Clapping.* Participants stands in a circle, hands held up as if just about to clap. They look at one other, until suddenly, without a hint or a signal, everyone tries to clap together. **This exercise encourages participants to listen attentively and practice "diag-red-nosis" (that is, the ability to translate information into action).**

3. *The Gibberish Circle.* Participants stand in a circle. One of them explains something in gibberish, and the rest of the group responds to or imitates the speaker. Everyone takes turns to be the speaker. **This activity helps to de-stress, have fun, listen to, and initiate the clowning interaction.**

4. *Birthdays.* Participants move about the studio, listening carefully. The moment the facilitator calls out a particular month of the year, all those born in that month begin to fall down while the remaining participants try to catch them before they hit the floor. **This is an exercise in active listening.**

5. *Opponent/Defender.* Participants stand in a circle. Each (mentally) selects someone as the "enemy" and another as the "shield." Each moves in a different direction in the room, always making sure to have one's protector between oneself and the "enemy." The group is in constant movement. **This is also an exercise in active listening.**

6. *"If ever . . .".* Participants stand in a room. One person announces something like, "If you've ever swum with dolphins . . . " Everyone who has swum with dolphins stands behind that person. You may tell a lie only twice (for example, to stand up and say such a thing even though you've never swum with dolphins). The participants continue making spontaneous announcements, although the "announcer" is always situated a little away from the group. **This activity enables the participants to develop rapport and enjoy the interaction.**

7. *Find the Differences.* Participants stand in pairs, facing each other, and decide who is Person No. 1 and who Person No. 2. Then Person No. 1 looks carefully at Person No. 2, how they seem to appear, their clothing, everything. They then turn around and stand back to back and Person No. 2 makes a change to a small detail in his appearance. When

they are face-to-face again, Person No. 1 has to identify the change. **This is an interesting exercise for active listening.**

8. *An In-depth Look.* Participants stand in two lines, facing each other. It is best that the pairs do not know each other. They will have to look into each other's eyes (at least from 1 to 3 yards away) but without dropping their gaze. The facilitator instructs the participants: come closer, draw away, turn and change places, hold hands, and so on. The participants have to follow the instructions but maintain eye contact at all times. **An exercise in empathy and building rapport.**

9. *The Hands Talk.* Participants are blindfolded. The facilitator forms pairs in such a way that no one knows who their partner is. Silence is maintained, and they are only allowed to "talk" with their palms, and create a "conversation" through the interactions of their palms. **This is an effective exercise in attentive listening, empathy, rapport, and improvisation.**

10. *"Everything we need is here."* Participants acts out a comical story using one another as substitutes for all the props and sets. **This is an exercise for group interaction using the language of humor and fantasy.**

B. EXERCISES TO DEVELOP ONE'S UNIQUE CLOWN PERSONA

Each participant must undergo a long, individual journey to discover one's inner clown. Their feedback is necessary on all issues and exercises in order to help and encourage the participant to discover and empower their individual clown persona.

1. *The Starting Point.* Sample exercise: narrate a true-life story as a clown, using clownish language (humor and fantasy).

2. *The Connection Point.* Sample exercise: tell a true-life story punctuated by imaginary clown-life stories, using clownish language.

3. *Costume Improvisation.* Searching for the unique clown character. Sample exercise: improvise with various clown costumes and interact with the other participants.

4. *Bodywork Improvisation.* Work on developing physical movement and expressiveness. Sample exercise: practice clownish aeronautics (that is, learn to fly under changing weather conditions).

5. *Facial Mimicry.* To develop the clown's mimicry capacities. Sample exercise: organize a contest for the most weird, frightening, or funny face. The winner is the participant with the most cheers from the audience.

6. *Objects and Puppets.* Certain props help the clown to develop skills in using objects, such as dolls and puppets. Sample exercise: storytelling with the help of an object to illustrate various aspects of the narrative.

7. *Voice Skills.* Voice training is imperative for the clown, as one has to constantly modulate and improvise. Sample exercise: participants should converse in pairs (while walking or sitting), changing their way of speaking (as the facilitator announces different situations using cue cards, if needed) in order to demonstrate various emotional expressions, volume, accents, and gibberish.

8. *Music.* It is also important for the medical clown to develop a keen interest in music and to be able to play at least one musical instrument. Music not only enhances the clown's performance but also plays a crucial role in the healing process. Sample exercise: participants could form a clown orchestra using various instruments, and work on their interaction. Musical activities are a great team-building exercise, and also help patients to identify with the clown and even participate in the performance.

9. *Humor.* Clowns should practice comic timing, and mannerisms, including various tropes like incongruence through polar opposites, exaggeration, reduction, and the

absurd. Sample exercise: clowns may choose to perform a specific form of incongruence, such as opposition, and build a gag based on the opposite gender or age (role-playing).

10. *Fantasy and the Poetic.* Clowns need to work on creating fantasy and poetry in order to develop their own repertoire and scripts. Sample exercise: form an imaginary clown universe using a roll of toilet paper (which becomes, say, a path over a chasm) and compose rhythmic gibberish verse to describe the shape of things in that environment.

11. *Gags and Improvisation.* Witty gags should be integrated in the improvised clowning interaction. For example, one may use some of the typical magician's gags and music, and combine and/or adapt them according to specific situations or locations (such as a waiting room, or a hospital ward, etc.).

12. *Time and Space.* The clown must develop site-specific work in spaces of varying sizes and over different time spans for various set of audiences. In other words, one should work on improvisation and clowning interactions for a small, crowded room as well for as a large hallway or a hospital ward with a few people isolated from each other.

13. *Simulations.* The clown should practice basic clowning interactions in hospital simulations and keep altering the basic conditions of the simulated space, as a hospital or even a makeshift medical facility is an extremely dynamic place of work. Sample exercise: the facilitator may instruct the participants to improvise an interaction with a child patient and the parents during a medical procedure while also conducting non-verbal communication with the nurse and physician.

14. *Structuring the Performance.* The clown must practice on building their performance from the time of entrance, the activity or interaction, until their exit. Sample exercise:

the medical clown enters a room, and gives a verbal explanation of everything in sight (the description allows the
facilitator to evaluate the medical clown's active listening),
continuing through to the "diag-red-nosis" (deciding on
the course of action).

Along with the practical hands-on training, it is necessary to have
a comprehensive, theoretical background of issues from the fields
of psychology, social work, expressive arts therapies, the history of
clowning, and anthropology. After the first stage of training, which
includes laboratory work in the studio on the fundamentals of
medical clowning and studying various aspects of theory, the second stage can commence: at this point, the beginner clowns
observe veteran clown doctors practicing at the hospitals (observing
them not as a medical clown but, rather, as a visitor). At the third
stage, the clown intern works for a period of time with an experienced medical clown who guides their learning and evaluates their
progress.

Before the beginner clown starts to work independently in a
specific hospital unit, the veteran clown introduces the new medical
clown to the entire healthcare staff (while privately describing the
work environment and the various personalities of the department),
During the initial period of work, it is desirable that the new medical
clown have a mentor for support and guidance, someone who will
observe, and from time to time, assist in the acclimatization.

Looking Forward: An Ideal Training Program for Medical Clowns

Most of the current training for medical clowns focuses on courses
on clowning language and the tools of humor and fantasy, practicing improvisation exercises and gags. The most correct training
would be intensive hand-on exercises that focus on all foundational
areas of medical clowning. In addition to the basic elements, an
important component in the work of a medical clown is the need
to cooperate with the medical staff. As a partner in an increasing

number of medical procedures, it is vital for the medical clown to be trained to work in tandem with the medical staff.

The knowledge of the psychology of the mental–emotional processes undergone by the patient and the patient's family, work and hygiene in the hospital and similar courses, will expand the medical clown's understanding and contribute to their practice. The medical clown must constantly update their skills through courses, seminars, and independent work. Due to the frequent encounters with terminally ill patients, death and suffering, inherent to the work and the unique bond created with patients, there is a high burnout rate despite the clowns' connection to pleasure and entertainment. The medical clown must seek therapy to restore the self after the pain from farewells, from suffering, and from the simple routine of work in a medical center.

CHAPTER SIX

Nurse–Physician–Medical Clown

A Model for Improved Teamwork in Medical Procedures in Pediatric Units

Medical clowns are now involved in many varied medical procedures, especially those for children, and studies have shown how their work contributes greatly to reducing anxiety among child patients (and their families) prior to and during these procedures. The triad of physician–nurse–medical clown is emerging as a new team model for many hospitals. This chapter analyzes this unique collaboration and proposes ways in which to improve the cooperation between this multidisciplinary team in order to benefit the well-being of child patients.

As I have already mentioned, medical clowning in public hospitals began in 1986 in New York with the collaboration of the Big Apple Circus's "Clown Care Unit" and the New York Babies and Children's Hospital. Over the next few years, the attendance of medical clowns in hospitals increased all over the US and the Western world. Most of the medical clowns are theater and circus performers who have adapted their performances to the hospitals and learned to cooperate with the medical staff. Many of the clowns are members of voluntary associations or organizations. They all have different criteria for bringing a medical clown on board and different training programs. These organizations are usually funded by donors and pay for the clowns' positions.

In 2006, the first academic program in medical clowning was launched in Haifa University, Israel, leading to a BA degree, with the collaboration of the Dream Doctors Project. The program included courses in theater and clowning on one hand, and nursing

NURSE–PHYSICIAN–MEDICAL CLOWN **79**

and psychology courses on the other. In recent years, the goal of the Dream Doctors Project has been directed toward professionalization in the field of Medical Clowning. Therefore, there is an increasing number of research studies on the subject and the Project is aimed at academic training of all of the Project clowns.

The presence of the medical clown within the healthcare system, as an integral part of the medical team, is neither to be taken for granted nor is it obvious. Over the last decade, more and more medical clowns have begun to take part, especially during medical procedures on children. At first, the medical clowns were brought in during routine tasks, such as taking blood samples, inserting IV lines, etc. But gradually they began to participate in greater number and were assisting across a varied range of treatments. It was clear, therefore, that a medical clown's presence in the treatment room was very helpful, since they could provide significant assistance in assuaging the child patient's anxiety and thus enabling the healthcare team (nurses and physicians) to carry out their work in an easier and smoother manner.

In recent years, researchers have reported on the medical clowns' important contributions to improving young patients' response to treatments and reducing fear and anxiety during the period of hospitalization.

The following case study illustrates the medical clown's practice, describing a female medical clown's intervention in a medical procedure: The clown was urgently summoned to the ICU where a 9-year-old girl had just been admitted with a deep cut in her foot. When the clown doctor arrived, the physician asked her to help in treating the girl, who was weeping as her foot was washed in an iodine bath. The clown immediately announced that she wanted a pedicure too (without really expecting any response from the nurse) and sat near the patient. To the clown's surprise, several minutes later, the nurse arrived with another iodine footbath for her. The medical clown removed her shoe and sock, and put her foot into the bath, just like the girl. The girl burst into laughter.

When the physician entered the room, the medical clown complained loudly that at last the pedicurist arrived, and that the nurse had not even offered them tea and biscuits while they waited. The patient continued to laugh, and slowly arrived at a state of relative calm. As a result, the patient's mother calmed down too; she whispered to the medical clown how lucky it was that she was with them. The physician requested that the clown accompany them into the "sewing room" where they would stitch up the girl's wound. When they entered the treatment room, the patient lay down on the bed, trembling with fear. But the medical clown was able to befriend her and to teach her a song in the time it took for the doctor to come into the room. The stitches hurt, and so the medical clown "threatened" the doctor that if he did not hurry, she would use her karate skills on him. The playful banter occasionally distracted the girl from her pain as she laughed and cried alternately.

Throughout the procedure, there was effective cooperation between the nurse and the physician and the medical clown, all of whom were working to reduce the girl's anxiety as well as her mother's fears. The clown was working as the child's ally, as if she was "defending" her against the physician, benefiting greatly in this from appearing different from the medial facility (which the child identifies as a system that causes pain), and thus enabling the formation of an immediate bond, a bond which alleviated the pain involved in the procedure.

Given the benefits, it may be useful to consider the ways in which the medical clowns' involvement may be expanded to a wider range of procedures while incorporating them into the multidisciplinary healthcare team.

The First International Conference on Medicine and Medical Clowning, the first of its kind, was held in Jerusalem between October 23 and 26, 2011, to mark the first decade of the Dream Doctors Project. The conference, attended by medical clowns from 22 countries, was primarily devoted to understanding and encouraging clown's participation in medical procedures. Senior physicians were also present to share knowledge on the issue. The discussion centered round a broad range of medical procedures, such as the presence of medical clowns while injecting botulinum toxin in children with cerebral palsy, with patients opting for in-vitro fertilization, during examinations for victims of sexual abuse, in treatment for patients of dementia, idiopathic arthritis, and PTSD, and medical clowning as a substitute for anesthetics during radio-nuclide scanning. These procedures form only a part of the broad spectrum of medical procedures in which medical clowns take an active part. Their presence in pediatric units is steadily rising, and it has been found that medical clowns are also present more often during dialysis and chemotherapy.

The manner and extent of the medical clown's involvement in a particular procedure result directly from, and are shaped by, two aspects: (a) the medical clown's capacity to assist the patient during the various medical procedures, impacted by the nature of the procedure and its implications for the patient; and (b) the interdisciplinary teamwork, nature and quality of the cooperation of the triad of nurse–physician–medical clown.

The Medical Clown Lessens Patients' Anxiety During Medical Procedures

Children and adults experience anxiety, pain, fears, and additional negative emotions before and during medical procedures. The following studies show that the medical clown assists in significantly reducing fears among child patients who must undergo a wide range of medical procedures. L. K. Hanson and his colleagues in 2011 explored, for over two years, the impact of the presence of a medical clown on children undergoing botulinum toxin injections in a hospital in Denmark. The research population comprised about 60 children who required repeated treatments, for a total of 121 procedures. The findings showed that the clowns' presence had a positive impact on treatments, especially when female medical

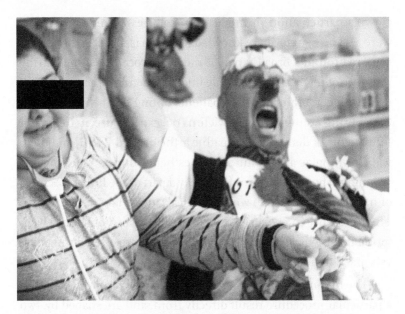

FIGURE 6.1 (ABOVE). The medical clown's performance reduces fear and anxiety during the period of hospitalization and improves child patients' response to medical treatments. Barzilai Medical Center, Ashkelon, 2009.

FIGURE 6.2 (BELOW). The clown reflects the patient's emotions through clownish actions, language, and gestures in order to express empathy. With a child patient at Barzilai Medical Center, Ashkelon, 2010.

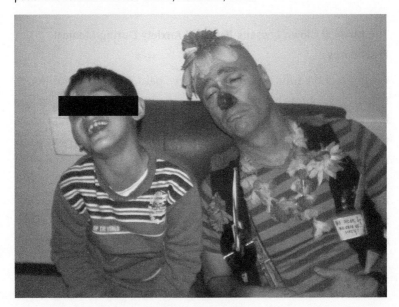

clowns were present during injections for girls. Certain procedures are likely to increase emotional trauma among boys and girls who have been sexually abused, since the procedures are invasive, designed to diagnose and treat, and often necessary in order for the findings to have legal validity.

In 2010, Dafna Tener and her team conducted a series of surveys and concluded that the presence of a female medical clown during medical examinations of sexually abused children significantly helped the children undergo the procedure more easily. The researchers stated that the children perceived the medical clown as their ally. It was noted that clowning alleviated the pain of the procedure for clown doctor activated dissociative mechanisms in the victims which facilitated suppression of the pain and distraction.

Children and their parents experience anxiety not only during procedures; the level of anxiety and apprehension rise the closer they come to surgical procedures. Studies, such as the one by G. Golan in 2009, have shown that when a medical clown accompanies the child into the operating room, anxiety is significantly reduced. When a medical clown remains with the child patient until the anesthesia is administered, their presence engages the child with positive interaction and good cheer. This helps balance the necessary health parameters before the surgery (blood pressure, heart rate, etc.) and therefore increases the chances of better recovery.

The study also found that anxiety becomes more intense the moment the anesthesia mask is placed over the child's face. The Dream Doctors addressed this precise critical moment and stated that they found a solution to children's discomfort with the anesthesia mask: they invented a game using the mask, with the child, before the procedure. The outcome is that the mask, even in the operating theater, is reduced to just one more prop for imaginative play.

Another study, led by Laura Vagnoli in 2005 and conducted on 40 children in Florence, Italy, showed that those who were accompanied by a medical clown had significantly reduced anxiety levels during pre-operative administration of anesthesia.

In situations of natural disaster or the crisis of war, many civilians suffer from shock and trauma. In such situations, the medical clown's intervention helps the physicians and counsellors in the health centers to treat PTSD patients. In the previous chapter, I have already described interventions by medical clowns with people suffering from PTSD who came to Barzilai Medical Center after rockets and mortar fire launched from the Gaza Strip from 2004 to 2008 by Hamas. The medical clowns were the first to assist in the Emergency Room, and succeeded in drastically reducing anxiety among children and adults suffering from shock.

Even in situations and procedures that lead to depression, not pain, especially among patients in deteriorated physical and mental conditions, the medical clown has a beneficial impact on their confidence and self-belief. In 2010, Orit Nuttman-Shwartz and his colleagues reported that the patients undergoing dialysis assisted by medical clowns at Emek Medical Center in Afula, Israel, showed remarkable improvement as opposed to others. Beyond lessening anxiety levels or improving the mood of the patients, the medical clowns had a positive impact on the results of certain procedures.

"Work Relations"? The Medical Clown as Part of the Multidisciplinary Healthcare Team

On the surface, the medical clown does not seem to be part of the multidisciplinary medical team in hospital. In most, if not all, countries, there is no official position mandated by any particular ministry of health. Usually the medical clown receives a salary as an outsourced service provider, without any medical liability, and for the most part, is not invited to participate in the medical staff meetings. However, according to the definition of teamwork, the medical clown is part of the multidisciplinary team and the clown must maintain work relations with other members towards their common goal—efficient and effective care of the patients.

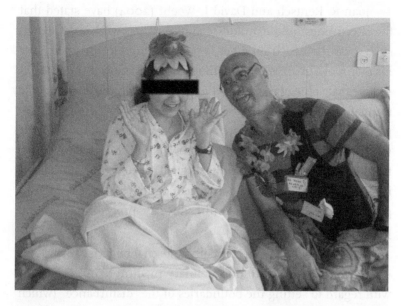

FIGURE 6.3 (ABOVE). Children perceive the medical clown as their ally. Chaim Sheba Medical Center, Tel HaShomer, 2011.

FIGURE 6.4 (BELOW). With a patient at the pediatric unit, Barzilai Medical Center, Ashkelon, 2010.

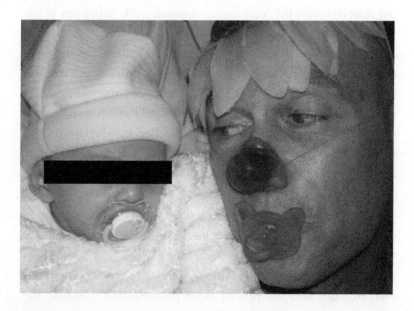

Joan R. Rentsch and David J. Woehr (2004) have stated that the effectiveness of the multidisciplinary team's work is defined in such a way that each member is perceived and in turn perceives his own work in accordance with the work of fellow teammates. It may be that some of the difficulties in the functioning of the triadic team of nurse–physician–clown lies in the other two professionals' perception of the clown's work as "mixing up" or "disrupting" their work, when in fact that is what empowers the child and helps the team by easing the child patient's fears. The clown's "disturbance" increases the child's willingness to gather up his own strength and give himself over to the painful, difficult procedure the child patient has to undergo.

The medical clown's difficulty and challenge is working in collaboration with a multidisciplinary medical team, especially with regard to setting the boundaries of the "disturbance" (which means setting the limits of the clown's performance only to enable effective diagnosis and therapy) or the "mix up" which helps in reassuring the patient and reducing anxiety and restoring a general sense of well-being, but in such a manner that the clowning does not interfere with the teammates' medical work. What lies at the foundation of this cooperation during medical procedures is, on the one hand, the space of the "disturbance" and "mix up" by the medical clown and, on the other, the professional space of the medical personnel. This is a very delicate balance, and rests entirely on mutual trust built over time and through familiarization and empathetic collaboration. As E. A. Glasper describes it, "The clowns [. . .] tread a thin line between legitimate parodying of the actions of the doctor or nurse, and 'ruffling the feathers' of malcontent" (2007: 27).

Iris Manor-Binyamini points to the lack of clarity referring to mutual expectations between the members of the multidisciplinary team as the major variable for the creation of conflicts. Working in a multidisciplinary team requires understanding not only one's own role but also the role of other professionals. Because the

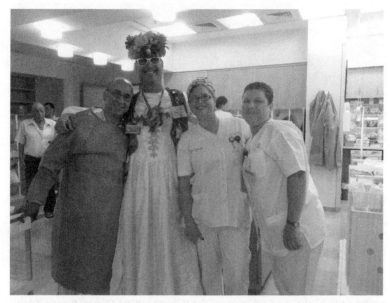

FIGURE 6.5 The clown and the medical team share a common goal, that is, to provide efficient and effective care to the patients. Rabin Medical Center, Petach Tikva, 2014. *Photograph by Hezi Panet.*

essence of the medical clown's work involves the unexpected, improvisation, and spontaneity, often breaking consensus and often provocative—the built-in lack of clarity in the medical clown's work is inherent in the attitude to mutual expectations in the multidisciplinary team—which are likely to lead to conflicts.

One of the major ways to bypass obstacles and avoid conflicts among the team members is to create a good communication system based on verbal and non-verbal communication, and to consider the role of emotional intelligence in influencing team effectiveness. It may be that of a consensual sign-language system between the medical clown, the physician, and the nurse, invisible or unintelligible to the patient, in order to prevent misunderstandings during the medical procedure. Good communication will also facilitate greater creativity; significant to the work of a multidisciplinary team that is especially meaningful for the medical

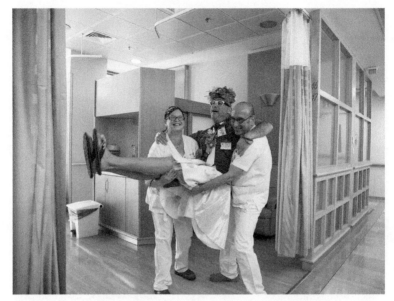

FIGURE 6.6 With the medical team at the Rabin Medical Center, Petach Tikva, 2015. *Photograph by Hezi Panet.*

clown, whose "performance" is, to a great extent, based on creativity and freedom of action. Having a medical clown partake in the multidisciplinary team during a procedure in hospital is no small challenge to some physicians and nurses who are experienced in carrying out those procedures for years without a medical clown alongside. They are now required to be flexible, to change the older work patterns, and to be able to adapt and act as one team—interdisciplinary teams must integrate the changing patterns and values with new modes of service delivery.

The interaction between the members of the multidisciplinary team and the patients in their rooms (and not only during medical procedures) is important since they are then more at ease. There is more space for the medical clown's "disturbance and mix up" in the rooms as well as more opportunities for mutual trust-building between all the parties. The medical clown's space of disturbance (playful disruption) and mixing up (role reversal, playacting, etc.)

is limited to the time of the medical procedures due to the professional intensity and concentration required by the treatment team
to administer the procedure, as well as the patient's pain and discomfort. But the interactions in the rooms on the ward are important too, because they serve as the foundation for the interaction
in the treatment rooms, conducted under conditions which are
more difficult. Consequently, the interactions in the patients'
rooms have greater impact on the work of the multidisciplinary
team during the medical procedures that follow.

Prof. Menahem Shlezinger, head of pediatrics at Barzilai
Medical Center, used to bring his entire retinue of doctors, nurses,
and residents into the patient rooms during his rounds. The medical clown nicknamed "Prof. Doctor Department Head" challenged
Prof. Shlezinger, claiming that he was the true head of the department and the professor an imposter. The respected professor
answered the challenge and a duel with sponge swords ensued,
accompanied by laugher of the children and the staff. The children
had to choose the winner. This loudly joyful cooperation between
the medical clown and the respected professor, witnessed by the
child patients, nurses, and doctors, had a tremendous impact in
the treatment room during later medical procedures. The children
who came for treatment that morning were calmer, smiling more
often, and responding well to their physicians when they saw the
medical clown standing near them, and the medical procedures
were conducted in a calmer way. The cooperation between the
medical clown and the team was better and accompanied by more
smiles than in the past.

N. J. Cooke and his colleagues (2004) have proposed a general
model for cooperation in a multidisciplinary team which can
become the basis for a specific model of the medical clown working
with the medical team. The first stage involves gathering data
for the task, the work, and the favorable group dynamics during
execution. The second is the processing of that data to generate
holistic knowledge for the team. The third involves the creation of

a holistic model for any given situation to lead to better execution of the task. Part of the first stage, according to this model, includes learning about and familiarization with the different roles and responsibilities of the other partners/team members. The medical clown must learn all of the details of the medical procedure and the routine that needs to be adhered to by all the partners for that specific procedure. It is similarly desirable for the nurse and the physician to familiarize themselves with the basic elements of medical clowning, because the medical clown usually has no set routine that can be "learned." In contrast to the other members of the team, who have a detailed protocol for carrying out a therapeutic procedure, the medical clown operates flexibly and intuitively according to the needs of the patient and in keeping with their physical and mental-health conditions. Learning about the basic principles of medical clowning is probably the best way for the multidisciplinary team partners to learn about the medical clown's sensitive practice.

Part of the second stage in this model may be to work toward developing a unique verbal and non-verbal professional language of communication between the clown and the team. During the third stage, the experts from the medical disciplines strive to create a joint work model for any given procedure which is flexible enough to adapt and contain the clown's creative and therapeutic "disturbances," facilitating the optimal execution of the physician's and nurse's work.

In recent years, medical clowning has entered a new era. No longer confined to the rooms in the ward, the medical clown is gradually becoming an integral part of the multidisciplinary healthcare team, and is involved in an increasing number of medical procedures carried out on children. Therefore, the need arises to create a new model of the multidisciplinary healthcare team's work to include the triad of nurse–physician–medical clown, based on the understanding of the necessary requirements for the effective execution of the procedures, clear instructions, and job definitions, and an agreement on the most desirable type of verbal and non-verbal communication among the team members. Such a model of work relations is likely to significantly improve the teamwork, as well as generate a more positive sense of well-being among the children and their parents during their medical procedures and period of hospitalization.

CHAPTER SEVEN

Medical Clowns Tell Their Remarkable Stories

In this chapter, I have selected 10 stories told to me by medical clowns during the interviews I conducted, and another four special stories that I was witness to. Some are extraordinary tales while the others are narratives from our daily routine at the hospital. All of them are from experienced medical clowns who have been working for years in various units in hospitals as part of the Dream Doctors Project.*

1. *I call this story, "The Pincushion." It made me laugh in surprise at the way the medical clown chose to maintain his place as a professional in the treatment room.*

After unsuccessful attempts to insert an IV line into his veins, the little boy whom the medical clown encountered seemed to look like a pincushion. The doctors and nurses kept trying to insert the branula even as the boy kept screaming at their every effort. Asked by the nurse to help the father hold his son down, the clown wiped the sweat off the child's brow while attempting to conduct a dialogue with the very upset mother standing in the doorway, unable to bear the sight of her son being pierced with the IV needle.

At this moment, a doctor walked in, a new one whom the clown had not met before, and asked the clown to leave the treatment room even though the clown had years of experience as an integral part of the pediatric medical-care team, and with great success. The clown responded that this was "his job" and that he would not leave the boy. Instead, the doctor could leave if he so

* Some names of patients have been changed to protect the privacy of the individuals.

wished; the clown would call in another. The parents began to laugh a this interaction, certain that this was a "staged" scene. The clown told the doctor, "So tell me what's easiest for you, and how I can best assist you, because I'm not going anywhere." The doctor had no answer. But the tension dissipated, the clown and the doctor smiled at each other, the boy and his parents calmed down as well and the procedure could thereafter be completed.

2. *The next story was told to me during one of my interviews. A medical clown found a way to bond with a teenage boy, hospitalized in a rehabilitation ward and then challenge him to do his physiotherapy exercises and not give up on himself. I call this one "The Wrestlers."*

The clown and the 14-year-old boy had a long history together, since the teen had been hospitalized in a rehabilitation facility for many months. The two liked to spar, with the clown pushing the boy from his wheelchair to the floor (but ever so carefully, so as not to hurt him at all), then tickling him until he "cried 'Uncle.'" Sometimes the clown and the boy would listen to music together, and sometimes they would watch Charlie Chaplin films.

During the physiotherapy sessions, however, the teenager turned out to be totally uncooperative and refused to budge from his wheelchair despite the physiotherapist's pleas. The clown then cut short the boy's excuses and "explanations" as to why he wouldn't get up, and told him, "Don't hand me that nonsense," and then begin to tickle him. Sometimes the clown would take the department's public-address system microphone and announce that the boy was a coward because he wouldn't get up. Of course, this would lead to another wrestling match. Finally, the boy would agree, and began to rise cautiously from his wheelchair, putting one foot ahead of the other, and then, accompanied by the medical clown, persevere with his exercises through the long months of rehabilitation.

3. *In "Facing Life," a medical clown was deeply affected by the distress of an adolescent boy whose face was disfigured by severe burns. Until the clown discovered how to empower the teen and give him hope in a way that went beyond the scope of his job—or did it?*

A 14-year-old boy had been trapped in a fire due to which his face was severely burned. The medical clown and the teen developed a friendship through their interactions in the burn unit, where the teen had been hospitalized for months. The friendship was a close one and they shared a great deal of laughter. But one day, the medical clown noticed that his friend was depressed, and had tears running down his cheeks. And he refused to tell anyone what he was sad about. The medical clown sat down beside him, waiting for to his friend to open us about his grief. "Look at my face!' the boy finally burst out, What kind of a life will I have? Who will marry me with a face like this? What's going to happen to me now?"

The clown tried to calm him down, to make him laugh and distract him, but nothing helped.

That evening, at home, the medical clown could not stop thinking about the boy. He felt he should do something over and above his usual attempts at good cheer, because the boy was in deep distress. So he went to his computer and did some research until he found three stories about people who had been disfigured in a fire and yet had gone on to succeed in life. All three had married, had children, had interesting jobs and full, happy lives. The clown printed out the stories and filed them in a binder. At their next meeting, he gave the binder to the boy and said, "You must realize that you have a future. Understand that the same thing happened to other people, and yet they are living happy, full lives."

The binder and the case studies helped the boy to gradually emerge from his depression and once again laugh along with the medical clown. The case studies and the continuing interactions between the clown and the boy gave the latter the strength and the motivation to address the difficulty and the pain involved in his extended rehabilitation process, and to confront his fears of the future.

4. Everyone makes mistakes. But this story from a superb medical clown who has been working for years tells of a mistake made very early in his career, the kind any beginner medical clown may commit due to lack of experience. This is the kind of mistake that can shape the medical clown's professional path. I call it "The Learning Experience."

A veteran street performer and actor, a clown who graduated from Jacques Lecoq's International School of Theatre in Paris but who was a beginner medical clown, began work at the pediatric emergency room (ER). One day, he entered the adult ER—where he was not authorized to be. One of the stations was concealed behind a curtain. The clown pushed it aside, and found the patient being examined by a doctor who immediately reprimanded the clown for entering a station even though the curtain had been drawn, and asked him to leave immediately. In response, the clown hugged the doctor with full-body contact while pretending to weep and winking at the patient. The doctor grew angrier, grabbed him by the arm and, shouting instructions to the nurses to keep all clowns out of the ER, pushed the clown out of the department.

This traumatic episode for the clown was a watershed moment in his career. Looking back, he said that he had crossed all possible lines simply out of a lack of understanding of the consensus or agreed-upon limitations to which the medical clown must always adhere. This was his first lesson in the necessary process of adaptation and understanding, from being an experienced street-theater clown into a medical clown.

5. We medical clowns create alternate realities through fantasy. Here is a story about a fantasy shared by a clown and a child patient that was so fascinating that it made reality disappear.

The story is about a 7-year-old boy with deep-seated anxieties. Terrified of clowns, the sight of the medical clown would have him screaming and suffering panic attacks. He also experienced similar anxiety attacks each time he had to undergo a medical procedure.

However, during the child's long hospitalization, the medical clown succeeded in slowly forming a bond with him and creating good communication and interaction. So that every time the child experienced a panic attack at the doctor and nurse trying to take a blood sample or press in an IV line, the medical clown was called in to assist.

One evening, the boy's mother called up the medical clown to remind him that the next morning the boy was scheduled for a procedure, and requested the medical clown to meet them in the treatment room. Usually the boy needed to be given a sedative, but that particular morning the medical-care team was going to attempt to carry out the procedure with only the assistance of the medical clown.

Through his acquaintance with the boy, the medical clown knew that he loved fairy tales and stories about fierce dragons and brave knights. The medical clown therefore began to improvise a play about a terrible dragon who could fly, spit fire, and who once attacked a village. As the medical clown acted out the dragon, he slowly moved into the treatment room, followed by the boy who couldn't stop listening. A woman physician awaited them in the treatment room, a doctor with excellent non-verbal communication skill and a high level of cooperation with the medical clown. She signaled to the clown that they should enter, and stood to one side. Acting out the dramatic fight between the knight and the cruel dragon, the medical clown succeeded in getting the boy to lie down on the treatment bed (without the violent physical struggle that usually broke out at this stage). The doctor prepared the needle and the equipment. The play reached its climax as the knight, narrowly missing the dragon's jaws, aimed his short sword at the dragon's heart. The medical clown maintained constant eye contact with the doctor who had already sterilized the area on the child's hand without him noticing. The clown timed the moment of the fatal stab with the moment the doctor was to insert the needle. At the decisive moment, the knight penetrates the dragon's heart with a deep, fatal thrust, and the dragon rolls over in the air, begins to shudder, loses control, and then falls lifeless to the ground.

When the dramatic story ended, and the boy realized where he was, he began to shout, "I don't wanna! Don't wanna!" The clown said, "You don't have to, nobody's doing anything to you, so let's get out of here." The procedure had been completed without the boy noticing anything at all, and the medication had been successfully administered without any difficulty.

6. *This is a story about "Magic Ice Pop." The clown tells of the illusion-creating soul and the clown's ability to transport a little girl to realms of imagination.*

A 5-year-old girl was lying in her hospital bed following a tonsillectomy. Since the surgery, her condition had deteriorated to the point where she could not stand up or even sit. The doctors could not diagnose her condition. The young girl was in a bad mood, so when the female clown came to visit, she grumpily told her mother to tell the clown to leave because she hated clowns. The clown told her she was quite right to dislike them—she couldn't stand them either. And then she turned to herself and asked herself to leave the room. Although, of course, she stayed.

The girl asked her mother to draw the curtain around her bed.

The medical clown stood outside the curtain and assured the girl that she was on guard and would make sure no one bothered her. "You can relax. I'll make sure no one comes in. I'll play you a tune to help you fall asleep."

But a doctor came along who wanted to examine the girl. It was a doctor who worked well with the clown. "You can't come in," said the clown, "I'm on guard here." The doctor asked the clown to check with the girl if was OK for him to enter. The clown went behind the curtain, and said to the girl, "There's a doctor here who wants to tickle you. Will you let him in?"

The girl found the situation very funny, and allowed the doctor to conduct the examination. The doctor helped her sit up but the second he let go, she slid to a reclining position for she had no muscle tone.

The doctor turned to speak to the girl's mother while the medical clown continued to interact with the girl: "Want to see what's in my basket?" The girl said yes, and sat up without any trouble. The clown glanced over to the mother and the doctor, wondering if they had noticed her sitting up. No, they hadn't. The girl was moving her legs energetically while examining the contents of the basket. Suddenly, she kicked the clown, who gave a yell, "Ouch!" The girl discovered a new game: she kicked the clown, the clown yelled, and looked sideways at the doctor and the mother. But they were so deep in conversation that they had not noticed what was going on. Then the clown asked the girl, "Want to come with me to buy an ice pop?" Of course she wanted to, but there was only one problem: she couldn't find her sandals. She called out to her mother a few times for her sandals, so she could go get an ice-cream with the clown. Only then did the mother and the doctor notice that she was sitting up and able to move her legs. The mother began to cry, said that it was indeed a miracle. The doctor couldn't believe his eyes while a young woman intern who had come in was looking at the scene with tears in her eyes.

The girl asked why her mother was crying, while the medical clown scolded everyone for distracting them from going to buy an ice. The sandals were strapped onto her little feet and the girl who had lain in bed, paralyzed, for weeks, got up and walked down the hall, holding the medical clown's hand, to go and buy an ice pop.

7. *This story features a creative medical clown who helps design "dreams to order" for children undergoing surgery. This is the story of "The Dream Machine."*

A 12-year old girl was sitting in the operating room (OR) waiting room, frozen in fear, a tense mother by her side. The female clown entered but did not make any eye contact; instead, she was busy inspecting her bracelets which she took out of her pocket. After a few minutes, it all became clear: she was a dream seller for those entering surgery.

The clown went over to the girl and asked her what kind of a dream she'd like to have during her operation. Where would it take place? Perhaps the beach, the pool or a park? Somewhere else? What would be the color of the dream?

The adolescent patient began to speak, and slowly the two of them, working together, wove the dream story. The medical clown clarified the specifics down to the last detail, each and every component of the dream. For example, should the French fries in the dream restaurant have ketchup or salt? Or mayonnaise or vinegar?

All of the details, of course, were written down with invisible ink on the bracelet the patient would wear when the order was complete. After she put on the plastic band, the girl was called in to the OR, accompanied by the medical clown. The patient lay down on the "Dream Bed" while the medical clown showed her the "Dream Machine" and explained how the dream would come through the pipe of the machine into the veins in her hand.

When the anesthetist came into the room—a doctor who was, of course, familiar with the procedure—the medical clown gave him the number of the dream and described its contents. The doctor commented, "No problem. It's a great dream," and promised to give it in a large dose. The 12-year-old girl looked amused, and very much at ease even as the anesthesia was about to be administered. When the process began, the medical clown came closer and repeated the details of the dream in a whisper into the girl's ears.

After she was "under," the medical clown took the mother by her hand and led her into the waiting room where they waited together until another girl came in, waiting for an operation and needing the clown to "sell" her a dream.

8. *A medical clown, who helps children undergoing painful medical procedures, told me the story of two Lumbar Punctures (LPs)—one successful and one unsuccessful . . . I narrate it in his voice.*

One day, I was called to substitute for a woman medical clown who usually works with the medical-care team carrying out Lumbar Punctures, a very painful procedure involving the insertion of a needle into the spine. The care team decided that it would attempt to carry out the LP without giving a sedative to the child patient. This seemed to me to be too great a demand on me, and I felt a great deal of pressure. The chances that I, as a medical clown, could replace the sedative seemed very slim to me, since the pain resulting from the procedure could be unbearable for a child. It felt like a heavy weight on me, and I felt that I was going into a situation with very small chance of success . . .

The team was composed of three nurses and two doctors whom I had not met before. It was also hot in the room—all conditions for failure. But in contrast to my low expectations, the procedure was completed with positive results. The child had no sedative but was fascinated by everything I did during our interaction. The reaction of the staff also seemed to "Wow! How did you manage to keep him so interested?!" The truth is that I can hardly remember what I did, but the boy was certainly involved with me for most of the time.

Unlike this case, there are unsuccessful ones. I remember the same painful procedure being carried out in the hospital I usually work at, where I know the staff. They did not sedate the patient, for they expected my clowning interaction to keep the young patient's attention off the pain. It began well, but at some point the pain was so great that nothing I did interested the patient, an adolescent boy. He went wild, and the doctors and nurses had to hold him down several times while his mother fainted. I wondered angrily how they dared to expect a clown to replace sedatives for such a painful procedure . . .

In such a procedure, the effectiveness of the medical clown depends on the level of pain the patient feels or can bear.

9. *Each patient and each situation is different, presenting a new challenge to the medical clown—which is why no solution can become routine. "The One-Time Magic Trick" tells of a small success.*

The head nurse asked the medical clown to visit Room 4, where a 10-year-old girl was refusing to take her medicines. He entered the room to see a very determined girl, her lips tightly shut, refusing to swallow the medicine from a syringe. But the medical clown had a bag of tricks, lots of little magical items. He had a small doll which could stand when he opened his palm. (He once showed me the trick: a little pin stuck into his palm; when he stretched out his hand, the little doll would stand up), or a coin which went into a bottle even though its mouth was smaller than the coin. He had lots of other tricks, which he performed for the girl but she could not be made to change her mind. The clown finally took the syringe, pasted a flower sticker onto it, handed it to the girl, and said goodbye. Just as he was about to walk out, the medical clown said, "Do you want to show me a little magic trick before I go, show me what you can do?" The girl drank the medicine down in one flash. The clown waved at her as he left.

"If you think this worked with other kids, you're wrong," he told me in the interview, with a big smile. "I tried but it didn't work. Next time I was called in on a case like this one, I had to find new ways to work with that child."

10. *Medical clowns are very skilled in improvisation and constantly adapting the healing performance to people and places. The clown's story describes an event of spontaneous collaboration between a medical clown and a doctor during a routine procedure undergone by a boy patient— who thought the whole thing was a game with "The Punching Bag."*

A young boy was sitting in the pediatric ER with his father, waiting to be examined by a doctor, when the medical clown walked in and then began a game with the boy, in which he threw brochures from a wall shelf onto the clown and she fell down while he laughed. A young doctor came in to examine the boy. She didn't know the clown, but quickly entered into the game. During the checkup, she also threw any object she could find at the clown. The clown tried to get up but every time something hit her, she "collapsed" to the loud laughter and joy of the little boy. The doctor continued her examination but the little boy hardly noticed. Usually the medical clown forms an alliance with the child patient "against" the doctors and nurses, but in this case, the "united front" was against the clown. The examination was soon over, but it seemed that the boy was willing to carry on so long as their game continued.

11. *The following are four stories drawn from my work in the oncology unit and hospice with adult patients with terminal illness. These encounters left me contemplating issues of chance, coincidence, and fate.*

i. *The "Telepathic Clown"*

One day, at work in the oncology day-care unit for adults, the nurse asked me to go over to a 40-year-old woman and try to lift her spirits. "Her name is Nogahut. See what you can do . . ." I was surprised at her uncommon name; it was the first time I'd heard it. The woman was sitting on a bed, her husband and mother in chairs near her. "Hi," I greeted her, "Could you just tell me your name . . . " I said, and closed my eyes, as if receiving telepathic messages. But before she could asnwer, I said, with clownish the-atricality, "Is your name Nogahut?"

"Yes, yes. The nurse told you. OK, thanks. Good you came over, but I'm fine. Now go and give some encouragement to someone who really needs it because I'm getting along fine, thank you."

"It's because you're a . . . " (once again I closed my eyes and spread my hands into the air) "psychologist?"

My guess was based on my experiences with several psychol-ogists.

"How did you know?" the mother asked, intrigued.

"My telepathic powers," said I, pleased at my accurate guess. "And I can also 'hear' that you are from . . . " (I mentined the name of a small rural village in the Negev). The mother was amazed, but Danny, the husband, provided the logical explanation (the correct one): "It's written on the bag there next to you."

Nogahut seemed amused.

"OK, let's see if you can name Mother's street in the village," she said, finally smiling. I closed my eyes again, and could see the village—not through my telepathic powers, but because my first girlfriend lived there, and I'd spent quite some time there. "OK, I see the entrance to the village (in my "medium's" voice, eyes still closed), and before me is the village square with three small frog statues. Maybe I should turn left here, right?" (I opened my eyes a crack and saw the mother nodding in surprise)."OK, the name of the street is . . . " (I named the street I knew that turns left from Frogs Square). And then I smiled into their amazed eyes. "OK, I can now go on to those who need me to amuse them . . . " (not that I really meant to leave just when I had "made contact").

"Wait a second, you're not going anywhere now," laughed Nogahut, curious to continue the game. "You didn't say where my husband and I live." I guessed again, ready to excuse my failure due to a foreign magnetic field which had entered the room and mixed up my telepathic powers. But, I named a city—simply because my father, returning to the country after many years abroad, had settled there. This time, I was no less surprised than the family with my guess.

But the best moment was when Nogahut asked me to name their street and I immediately named the only street I knew—the one on which my father lived. They did indeed live on the same street! This extraordinarily strange "coincidence" marked the beginning of a long, close relationship with Nogahut and her family. (Of course, I was never tempted to have another telepathic session with them, so as not to ruin the strong impression of our first encounter).

Whenever we met during her long course of chemotherapy, we laughed and had a great time. The three of us used to sing, as it turned out that Danny loved music and could play the harmonica. Of course, my trusty guitar would always come along. And I would dance with Nogahut's mother, Lily.

Unfortunately, the treatment did not cure her, and about a year later, Nogahut's condition deteriorated. One day I saw her in the lobby, her face in her hands and sobbing. Her mother was sitting next to her. When her husband saw me approaching, he told me in sign language that it was a bad time. Several weeks later, I ran into her, and saw that her face and neck were very swollen; I recognized it as a side effect of the large dose of steroids given to cancer patients to lessen the pain.

When we met last, she was eating a sandwich with great appetite, and said nonchalantly that she wanted to say goodbye to me. I asked her where she was going, and she said, "I guess you lost your telepathic ability." She was not going on a trip but going to die. The doctor had said she had a few weeks left, so she would not be coming in for any more treatments. She looked at her mother and said she hoped to live until the summer because she wished for the whole family to go on vacation together. Her mother nodded, silently.

I shook Nogahut's hand and thanked her for all of the laughs we shared. She admitted that she had been mistaken at our first meeting: she did indeed need me, and thanked me for accompanying her on her journey. We said goodbye to each other, and I parted from her for ever.

What should a medical clown do when he doesn't really feel like going to work? This is what happened to me one special day:

ii. The Clown's Birthday

One evening, I was wondering whether or not to go to work the next day since it was my birthday. It would be a great idea, I thought, if the family could go on a hike or celebrate in some special way. The next morning, I decided that I would go to work as usual, but do something special after work in honour of the day.

The moment I entered the oncology ward, Dalia, the secretary, informed me that the hospice had phoned the desk and asked me to help celebrate the birthday of one of the patients. That's strange, I thought to myself, I've been working in this department for two years, and this is the first time the hospice called up and asked me to come. And it was the first time I had been asked to help celebrate someone's birthday—and that too one on the the same day as mine. Many philosophical thoughts passed through my head while I made my way to the hospice building, thoughts about serendipity, fate, and chance. Was there really such a thing as coincidence?

When I arrived, the doctor who was the hospice director greeted me along with the patient's family, and they all told me a bit about Edith. These were her final hours. She had been given painkillers and sedatives but was aware of her surroundings. I asked how old she was and it turned out that she was my age.

I entered the room playing birthday tunes on my guitar and the family followed with a cake and balloons. As we sang, "And one more to grow on for next year," Edith's mother could no longer hold back her tears, and Edith's husband's voice cracked with emotion. I sang and danced with the family while Edith smiled a weak, sad smile of farewell. Later I went over to her bed and sang quiet, songs to her, songs I invented, songs that told her how much her family loved her. I celebrated *our* birthday. And before I left, I was warmly hugged by her family.

When I left the hospice, I looked up at the heavens and took a very, very deep breath . . .

iii. *"A Moment of Happiness in the Geriatric Ward"*

Department E at Hartzfeld Geriatric Hospital is the "last stop' for many chronically ill adults. Many of the elderly patients I met there had been hospitalized for long periods, from a few months to several years, and a large number of them ended their lives in that ward, many suffering from dementia in various degrees of severity.

Georgette was one such patient, about 90 years old, with advanced dementia. Born in France, she'd lived there for many years but now mostly sat in a wheelchair in the lobby, wearing a lost and sad expression. Sometimes she'd call for the nurse in a mix of French and Hebrew. Her daughter came to visit her every afternoon but she, too, was sad because Georgette could not always recognize her or communicate with her.

On that particular morning, I saw Georgette seated on a chair, her daughter looking sadly at her. I went over and asked Georgette, "Would Mademoiselle like to hear a song?" When she failed to respond, I repeated the question even louder, but there was still no answer. I began to hum "Autumn Leaves" ("Les feuilesmortes") by Yves Montand, and slowly Georgette opened her eyes wide and began to sing along. Her daughter sang along too. "She remembers the words!" the daughter exclaimed in disbelief. A huge smile spread over both faces as Georgette continued to sing, her eyes glowing. Her daughter held her hand and a tear ran down her cheek while I strummed along on the guitar. I was quite moved by the moment of grace that I could help create between mother and daughter. One week later, Georgette fell into a coma, a terminal "twilight state" and no longer communicated with anyone.

The last story in this chapter tells of the beginning of the relationship between a medical clown and a man with a terminal illness.

iv. *"Stairway to Heaven"*

One morning at the oncology day unit, Nurse Penina gestured to me to step closer to her desk. Clearly, she had something to tell me. When Penina looks stern and beckons me to come over, I know that one of our patients has passed away. "It's Efrem," she whispers, and my heart misses a beat. In my mind's eye I could see his broad, smiling face. Effi was a "man of large proportions," always optimistic and in good spirits, sensitive, with a rumbling voice, and cynical humor. I remember our first encounter which took place months ago. I stood at the doorway with my red nose, bubblegum-pink fake eyeglasses, fabric flowers sprouting from my head, flowery trousers, colorful shirt with a vest and tie, my chest proudly boasting a variety of medals and seashells and several name-tags, among them "Prof. Dr. Department Head," another with the slogan, "Vote for the *ZeinGesunt* (Be Healthy) Political Party," yet another stating "Single man seeking a match," and on the fourth, in mirror-writing, "What do you care what this says, Noseybody." My guitar hung on its shoulder strap. Effi was lying on the bed, the chemotherapy cocktail flowing into his arm through an IV drip. He looked me up and down, grinning, his wife Michal by his side. "OK, let's see if you can play me some Jethro Tull," he challenged me. I began to sing a cut from *Aqualung*, and he joined in right away. This was the beginning of our interaction. For months, we sang songs form rock bands we both loved.

After he passed away, I visited Michal during the week of mourning at their home in Rishon LeZion, and she told me that she had noted down all the songs Effi had asked me to sing with him. They formed the "playlist" for his funeral. Effi was buried to the sounds of Led Zeppelin's "Stairway to Heaven."

CHAPTER EIGHT

"Oh Yeah, about Those Clowns"

Physicians, Nurses, and Other Medical Care Personnel Talk
About the Medical Clowns

As part of my research on medical clowning, I interviewed 63
physicians, nurses, and paramedical professionals (physiothera-
pists, occupational therapists, and others) working across seven
pediatrics departments, two internal medicine wards, two oncology
wards, surgery and rehabilitation (and another three units: emergency medicine, outpatient day center, and intensive care) at
Chaim Sheba Medical Center and Barzilai Medical Center. The
interviews explored the work of medical clowns under the aegis
of the Dream Doctors Project, especially those who have been
working with medical professionals and paramedics over the past
decade.

The majority of the medical staff expressed deep appreciation
for the work of the medical clowns, but there were other opinions
as well. In these semi-structured interviews, I attempt to examine
the medical clowns' work as an integral part of the medical-care
team during various medical procedures, and as perceived by the
medical-care staff members. I wanted to present case studies of
both successful and not-so-successful collaborations.

The following quotations are all extracted from my recordings
of these interviews.

A Nurse in the Pediatric Oncology Unit: "Four physicians were having
a serious discussion when a medical clown entered the ward and
began to make a tremendous racket. One of the doctors became
quite irritated and asked her to tone it down. The medical clown
apologized, and then apologized again, about 8 more times. It

made everyone laugh. The spirit of foolishness is a great thing. I envy them. It changes the atmosphere in the department. About 90% of the time it's the coolest thing in the world, but 10% of the time I have to tell them 'it's not a good time now'."

A Nurse in the Pediatric Internal Medicine Department: "There was a 3-year-old boy in the burn unit who was suffering from 15% burns. Treatment was very painful, despite the sedatives. But the clown gradually developed a friendship with him and succeeded in making the boy like her. He was so fascinated by her that he didn't let out a peep right through the treatment. She succeeded in diverting his attention totally, which was amazing."

A Blood Technician in the Pediatric Oncology Unit: "I have worked with many clowns in recent years. There is a short procedure of taking blood, it takes a minute or two. Before, I had a negative image of clowns. But here I've met clowns who are educated, charming people, and I have grown quite close to them. They help me when I take blood samples, work side by side with me. And the children find it easier to undergo the procedure with them around. The clowns know how to work quietly with me because I can't stand noise. It's bad enough when the children yell at being pricked with the needle. If any other noise is added to that, it's too much for me."

Hemato-oncology Physician I: "Full disclosure: I don't like clowns. Ever since I was a little girl, I have not liked them. They don't make me laugh, or calm me down—they only make me nervous. And, amusingly, the same goes for my kids. At work, the clown did help some children cope with treatments and hospitalization, but perhaps not very much. Sometimes the clown annoys me, especially when they make too much noise. Sometimes, even here in the room, you could be trying to talk to someone, and right outside there's chaos—lots of children, and then the clown (especially female clowns) screaming with a fake joyfulness . . . I don't think these screams are beneficial. There are unwritten hospital rules, for example: no running and no shouting, because people run and shout in an emergency. So, OK, they come and make a happy scene, but sometimes it's just too much."

Hemato-oncology Nurse I: "Two cases come to mind: one was a successful intervention in which an 8-year-old girl donated bone marrow to her brother. The medical clown entered the room and the girl enjoyed the performance extremely, and the procedure went well. But, there was another case in which a 17-year-old girl and her mother asked the medical clown to leave because it was inappropriate for them at the time, and the medical clown politely left the room."

Hemato-oncology Nurse II: "I have had good experiences with clowns both as a mother and as a nurse. When my son fell ill and was undergoing treatments, and I could not calm him down, the clown with her songs and a small noisemaker succeeded in diverting his attention. In general, I think that a medical clown's work is harder than my work as a nurse. I'll have to carry out the procedure even if the child screams, but to stand there and make the child stop screaming, even make him laugh and smile, requires a special talent."

Hemato-oncology Nurse III: "The medical clowns are good for the medical-care staff. Sometimes there's tension and they 'puncture' the 'heavy' atmosphere. I'll never forget how, once, one of the senior physicians came over to the ward with a senior doctors from abroad. The atmosphere was so tense, so serious. Then one of the medical clowns came by, as if to shake hands, and said, 'Nice to meet me, nice to meet me!' That eased the tension and everyone became quite jovial."

Pediatric Surgical Nurse I: "A successful case story: I was taking a blood sample from a 3-year-old girl who was screaming. A medical clown came in and almost immediately succeeded in calming the toddler and making her focus instead on the soap bubbles she was blowing and the puppets she activated. This helped me complete the procedure, and I was very glad the clown was with me. I also have a story of a case which did not succeed: a family had just been given the news that their son had a cancerous tumor in his head. They were sitting in shock, the little boy crying. A medical clown who was unaware of the situation came in, and it wasn't suitable. I had to ask her to leave, and told her about the case when we were outside."

Hemato-oncology Physician II: "I have no objections, but I have no need for medical clowning. I never saw huge successes, never saw medical clown change a situation 180 degrees. But, yes, their presence is somewhat nice, it amuses the kids, it brings a momentary smile to their faces. It's sweet, but it seems to me less meaningful than, say, a social worker or art therapist.

For example, a boy who was crying because he was frightened of a blood test—I didn't see a medical clown convincing him to go through it. I didn't see that. A boy who was anxious before a procedure remained anxious. Or a little girl who was sad. The medical clown came in, then played with her and she laughed—that was nice. But two hours later she was sad again. So it didn't bring about any fundamental change. I wouldn't say that clowning is unnecessary, but it has a slight effect, less than that caused by the presence of other therapists.

When I'm in the treatment room, and a medical clown comes in, it makes me feel a bit under pressure. I feel I'm in a situation in which I have to participate in the amusement. And I'm not sure that I'm amusing or amused. Maybe there are expectations of me, expectations of something I'm not sure I can provide. Sometimes it even annoys me. For example, once I was standing near a child's bed, trying to speak with him, and there was a problem, and just two yards away there were bells ringing, honking sounds, someone jumping about—all of which were driving me crazy. Here was something I needed to concentrate on but there was chaos on the other side of the room. I had to shout and try very hard to listen to the patient. I found the clown's ruckus rather disrespectful. It irritated me."

Hemato-oncology Nurse IV: "We had a case of a 4-year-old boy who had a problem with his hand. We were trying to get him to move it. For days he refused. Then, when the medical clown arrived, through his games and soap bubbles, he succeeded in getting the boy to move his hand. It was amazing. Later, the parents adopted the medical clown's methods to help keep their son's hand active."

A Nurse in the Internal Medicine Ward I: "I have been on the job since the past nine months. There's a medical clown on the ward who's an 'old-timer' and I frequently go to her for advice. Not long ago, we had a terminally ill young girl in a separate room with her mother who was, naturally, very sad. I consulted with the medical clown who helped me with advice about how I could strengthen the mother and make the girl smile a bit. There was another instance: I wasn't confident enough with certain procedures. I was treating a baby who was screaming and resisting the procedure. The medical clown entered the treatment room and performed a pantomime—the baby stopped screaming and began to stare at him. That helped me very much to connect the transfusion."

Pediatric Surgical Nurse II: "This happened just now: a 3-year-old boy with hemophilia, from whom I had to take a blood sample, was screaming. But when the medical clown came into the room he began to laugh, because only a few minutes ago they had been playing in his room. His memory of their game was still fresh. They picked up from where they had left off, and he forgot about the examination. But there are other children who are afraid of the medical clowns and request that we not let them in the room."

A Nurse in the Pediatric Internal Medicine Department: "I remember a baby being treated in the burn unit who was so fascinated by the medical clown that he didn't make a sound. I also remember a different case of a boy with burns, screaming. His parents were on edge and asked that the medical clown leave because he wasn't helping at all."

Pediatric Internist and Emergency Medicine Unit Physician I: "I have a positive opinion of medical clowns. For the most part they assist me in my work, but there are some cases in which the clown interacts with the child using his guitar and his music in such a way that I am unable to conduct the examination and this holds me up unnecessarily."

Hemato-oncologist II: "It's difficult for me to talk with the medical clowns when we're not in front of the children. They remain clowns—you can't talk to them like regular people. I understand that we are colleagues and that we can talk, but I don't want to hear honking from your red nose right now. It disturbs our communication."

Internist and Pediatric Emergency Medicine Unit Physician II: "I am very much in favor of medical clowns, and think that every doctor has to be a clown while examining child patients. You have to talk to them at their level and often be silly. The feedback I receive from parents is that I appear to be half-doctor and half-clown which, I believe, is a compliment. I stoop to the patient's eye-level and move my body in a funny way to make children and their parents laugh. I've adopted a method to treat the children, part of which I've learned from the medical clowns: with toddlers, I use colors and sounds to make contact; and with older children, I talk about superheroes. I get into their world. If I were head of the department, I would encourage the doctors to clown around more often with the children. I have a new idea: to have medical clowning training for the doctors. Most of them finish the work day not with the greatest feeling or motivation. It seems that the medical clowns could be there for them too, to make even them feel better."

Pediatrician I: "I am divided on my opinion of medical clowning. On the one hand, I have seen how it helps in several cases. On the other, there are children who are afraid of clowns. As for me, the noise they make is very disturbing. I try to hint that it's disturbing the procedure but they don't always understand. It's as if they have no limits. I assume it depends on the particular medical clown, but sometimes it's just too much. I remember one examination, of a very small baby who was screaming. The medical clown made a great deal of noise without realizing the gravity of the situation. I tried to hint gently because I'm not an assertive person, but it didn't help. The patient was an infant, and the mother felt extremely anxious. She was trying to tell me something but it was impossible to talk because of the noise the medical clown was making."

Pediatrician II: "I think that when there are medical clowns working in the department, parents feel they're receiving better medical care, and they're right. I distinguish the differences between the medical clowns: some work wholeheartedly while others less so. A medical clown who's not really enjoying their work to the fullest or participating wholeheartedly should find another job."

Pediatric Internist and Emergency Medicine Unit Physician III: "In my experience, medical clowning always works. It makes the kids feel special, and helps me as a doctor to carry out procedures effectively."

Internist and Emergency Medicine Unit Physician: "The medical clowns succeed in calming the child patients, and even making some of them to smile and laugh, at least 70% to 80% of the time that I am taking blood or inserting an IV line. In a minority of cases they do not succeed because of the child's extremely high level of anxiety. I have never been in a situation in which a medical clown disrupted the treatment in any way."

Physiotherapist I: "The medical clown helps me greatly when I need to take measurements for the pressure suit for burn victims. The clown diverts the patient's attention and make it possible for me to complete the task efficiently because the measurements have to be extremely accurate. He helped me, for example, when the child had to move his hand: the clown performed the movement and the child imitated him. But on one occasion, the clown seemed to interrupt the procedure—when the boy had to do some cognitive work and I had asked him all sort of questions, the medical clown quickly gave the answers instead of the child."

Physiotherapist II: "The medical clowns make me laugh a lot, and I'm amazed by their creativity. One day, in the intensive care unit, there was a boy in a very serious condition—he could not move his limbs. While interacting with him, the medical clown took the sterile coats (used by medical personnel) and built a kind of tent over his bed. She succeeded in having him smile and respond. Several doctors who saw the coats hanging above a bed—a strange and unusual sight—became nervous and rushed over to understand the weird display. When they got there, they all began to laugh. That morning I envied the medical clown's creativity in her interaction with the boy."

Physiotherapist III: "I was treating a 2-year-old boy who refused to walk. He would scream and resist the walking exercises. When the medical clown arrived, the child began to cooperate; he followed the medical clown, walking. It is reasonable to assume that at that point the treatment seemed to him like a game."

Pediatric Internist: "The medical clowns are not always available, and are here for a little while. Some are more successful than others. I think medical clowns have to be aware about medical procedures and be involved in them. They have to love children as well. There are some medical clowns who love children and love their work, but I feel there are others who force themselves to do it. Some medical clowns try to win over the child and try all sorts of things while others attempt one thing. And if the child cries or resists, they give up—if a child refuses to cooperate, the clown makes no effort whatsoever. There's a type of medical clown who will blow up balloons and sing funny songs and the child will laugh and cooperate—then it's nice to be working in such a fun atmosphere. But there are other types of medical clowns who will come in, try to make funny noises—but lack patience. That kind of clown, who lacks the desire to see the child happy, will quickly despair. That's the difference as I see it. I feel that there are some clowns whose heart really isn't in their work."

Hemato-oncologist III: "I'm very much in favor of medical clowning, I think it has a very important function—it improves the entire atmosphere. The child patient enters the procedure with fewer fears and tears, especially if he becomes familiar with it before it even begins. When a patient enters the treatment room with the medical clown, it breaks down all the mental walls they have built up about the procedure. It makes it possible to proceed in a more pleasant way, with a bit of laughter and good humor. Of course, this is not always the case. But yes, the clowns make it possible for children to view their treatment in a more fun way because they divert their attention."

Pediatrician IV: "Overall, I think that medical clowning is an excellent practice, but not always appropriate. I've seen really incredible cases. For example, during sedation in a burn treatment. Even after we administered the drugs, the medical clown with her music was the one who succeeded in calming the little girl and putting her to sleep. In contrast, sometimes it's not the right thing to do, or it may not work. For example, there was a medical clown here who started to talk about food and cakes right near an anorexic girl. You have to understand the situation: who is around you, and what are they sensitive about. In that case, the medical clown wasn't familiar with the situation. So they need to be briefed before they visit a patient. Nevertheless, it's usually very successful. There are clowns with whom it's easier for me to work; I think it's entirely a matter of personal 'chemistry.'"

Pediatrician V: "I think that good medical clowns can ease the atmosphere in the room, not only for the children but also for the parents and the medical staff. I have a dialogue for cooperation during the examinations with the medical clowns I've known for several years; with the new ones, it's more like a performance you see from the side. I feel comfortable working with the medical clowns I've known for a long time. I can't remember a clown ever having bothered me in any way. There are some clowns who 'perform' and others who blend themselves into the situation, making it easier and more comfortable for me to work with them. As I see it, medical clowning has a very positive effect."

Pediatric Internist and Intensive Care Unit Physician: "In my opinion, the medical clowns should work in the hospital every day. I would even take them to my clinic. They make our work easier, and it gives us the opportunity to have a calmer and quieter child patient who cooperates better with us. The medical clown's game, the toy, the story, etc., remain in the child's mind for a very long time. I can tell you about a girl who was in an extreme state of anxiety during a war. It was only thanks to the presence of a medical clown that she was able to lessen her anxiety and this in turn made it possible for me to examine her."

Pediatric Internist II: "At first, when I started work in the department and the medical clown would pass me by with her monkey puppet. I would pretend that the monkey bit me. Then she told me that frightened the children. Since then, we have learned to work together, to go with the flow during the games in front of the children. This has implications for everyone, even the parents, who see that there are friendly relations across the ward. It's not like: oh, here's the doctor, and here's the medical clown, and each one is doing the work without any connection to the other. But that there's a nice relationship between them. That makes everyone feel better.

I think it's important to create a personal bond with the medical clown, and for the medical-care team to be familiar with the clown's work. I sometimes hear negative reactions from doctors who say they don't want the clowns in the treatment room because it disturbs their work. There are younger doctors who feel pressured, and the presence of a medical clown in the treatment room makes them feel that there's another pair of eyes examining them, even disturbing their concentration. But there are also some experienced doctors who prefer that the medical clown not enter the treatment room."

A Nurse at the Internal Medicine and Pediatric Intensive Care Unit: "Many of the children come in for repeated hospitalizations. They know the staff and the medical clowns, and when they arrive, they ask about which medical clown is working that day. They await them eagerly. The relations between us and the medical clowns in the department are so good that once I telephoned her, on my own, in the afternoon, because I had a little girl patient in a state of tremendous anxiety. The medical clown came in especially for her; this established a sense of trust between us. The medical clowns should be available and accessible, as they are part of the medical-care team. This is a multidisciplinary job, and there are many times when we were unable to do the task without the medical clown's timely interventions. She contributes so much to what we do. She has become part of the team even outside of working hours; she's on our WhatsApp group and joins us often for social events. A medical clown has to be part of the care team."

A Nurse in the Internal Medicine Ward II: "My son who was hospitalized in the orthopedic ward 3 years ago—he is 9 years old now—remembers only one thing from that time: the medical clown. He doesn't remember how much it hurt, how he had to lie there with his arm tied in a raised position—he only remembers the medical clown. He still asks me how Prof. Doctor, the medical clown, is doing, the one who came over to him with his green frog and finger puppet. Every day he would wait for the clown to visit. Every day he was in hospital, he would wait, and ask, "Mom, when is Prof. Doctor, the Clown, coming? I have fun with him. He's so nice and happy." The medical clown had a finger puppet called Esther who would jump around and bump into the wall. That really made my son laugh. Then there was the talking green frog, and the pacifier the clown would suck on like a big baby, which was all very funny to him. All of the very individual interactions with the boy, in the many languages the medical clown spoke, the Russian song—which is what my son listened to at home—would "take him home," calm him down and make him feel at home even though he was very, very far away from home. My experience of the medical clowning as a mother preceded my experience as a nurse, and it was always very positive. It made me laugh as well, and I saw my son happy. What could be better than that? It reduced my fears. It was a very positive change. Later on, I experienced the medical clowning work as a nurse, and I feel it works wonders."

A Nurse in Pediatric Internal Medicine Ward I: "I'm new here, I've only been here a year,. The medical clowns who come in with me to carry out procedures take the pressure off me, so I can concentrate more on what I'm doing. The child patient focuses on the clowns' performance, and I don't have to face resistance during the procedure—while taking a blood sample, or inserting an IV line. It helps me very much because I'm constantly under pressure to work with care, and I have to concentrate very hard."

A Nurse in Pediatric Internal Medicine Ward II: "I am personally acquainted with the medical clown. I like to cooperate with her and give her space. I pay attention to the child patient and their needs, and want them to have a better experience of care. The clown and I have a close friendship and I can sense her mood, so I know what and how much she can do on any given day."

CHAPTER NINE

Patients Fight for "Their" Medical Clown

This chapter chronicles the struggle by inpatients and outpatients diag-
nosed with cancer, their families and friends, in one of the largest med-
ical centers in Israel, protesting the dismissal of "their" medical clown
due to budget cuts. Their protest against the hospital administration
took place in April 2014.

The protest gave rein to the patients' feelings, demonstrating the
vital importance of the interaction between the medical clown and adult
patients coping with a major illness. Beyond the saga of a particular
individual, this event depicts the professional position of the medical
clown in the hospital as the first employee to be fired during financial
difficulties, despite the patients' feeling that medical clowning effectively
alleviates their pain and is an essential component for their recovery.

For years, medical clowns have been working in various pediatrics
units at a medical center in central Israel as part of the Dream Doctors Project. In April 2012, a veteran medical clown (let's call him
"Dr. Clown") was asked for the first time to work with adults in the
oncology department at the same medical center, with outpatients
at the day clinic and with hospitalized patients. The hospital administration was persuaded to introduce the medical clown in medical
teams caring for adults, despite the great skepticism felt (and
expressed) by some medical professionals in the department. The
doctors asked the medical clown not to make too much noise and
to avoid playing his guitar, and gave him a long list of other caveats.
Of course, being a clown, Dr. Clown immediately agreed to everything and then went to do just the opposite (although, as a trained
medical clown, Dr. Clown was well aware of the nuances of
patients' conditions and their ramifications).

Very quickly it became clear that the hospitalized adult patients as well as the outpatients needed a medical clown no less—and perhaps even more—than the child patients. However, in April 2014, the hospital administration removed positions and restricted working hours for the medical clowns in the pediatric units, though leaving quite a few still on the job. In contrast, they decided to terminate Dr. Clown's employment in the adult units, leaving them without any medical clown in their department—and this led to a dramatic and entirely unprecedented struggle . . .

Although Dr. Clown knew that his encounters with the patients were meaningful, he had no idea about the depth of their signifi-cance. Nor did he expect the intensity of the reaction. As soon as they learnt of the decision to fire "their" clown, the patients organ-ized themselves through social media, e-mails and phone trees. They drew up a letter to the hospital administration requesting immediate cancellation of the decision, and describing how impor-tant the medical clown's work was to the patients being treated in the various oncology units or hospitalized in the ward. Several dozens of patients, their families, and friends signed the letter:

The e-mail to Head of Research Fund and other senior members of the staff at the hospital, copied to specialized medical and health-care associations

To: Head of the Research Fund, Hospital,
Deputy Director, Medical Center
Ombudsman's Office, Hospital

From: Patients, Families, and Friends

Re: Request from patients regarding the termination of employment of Dr. Clown—Medical Clown in the oncology departments at the Medical Center

We, the undersigned, inpatients and outpatients at the Medical Center, oncology clinics, and departments—and our families—are requesting you to cancel the harmful decision made to terminate the employment of Dr. Clown, the medical clown who entered our lives and is accompanying us with love during this difficult period of our lives.

Research studies examining the issue of medical clowning point to the positive impact on patients' coping process and recovery. Signs of these findings can be found in the academization of the field and the establishment of degree programs in this discipline.

However, we are now writing this letter not as people attempting to study the field academically, objectively, and from afar, but as patients and patients' families and friends who have directly experienced Dr. Clown's significant impact on the processes of coping and recovery in the oncology departments and the oncological day clinic at the Medical Center.

It seems unnecessary to explain to you the great suffering, pain, tension, and anxiety accompanying cancer. All of these are clear even to those who have not experienced it, and surely to those who have experienced curative treatments. It is utterly surprising to hear about the decision to fire Dr. Clown who makes hospitalization and treatments more bearable, whose presence is the only point of light in this darkness of great intensity. We cannot imagine you extinguishing this light and its power to heal and alleviate suffering.

It is hard to decide where to begin to describe the Doc's contribution: many patients make their appointments for treatment and time according to Dr. Clown's schedule. How he eases our distress as we wait for blood tests, treatment, and medications is truly and concretely felt. Dr. Clown's unique personality has enabled him to establish an intimate, emotional bond with patients and their families alike. His commitment and his desire to give, his sensitivity and ability to reach out to each patient, his music and improvisational talent, succeed in eliciting laughter from the patients (even from the skeptics and cynics among us).

Moreover, many times, it has seemed that amid all of the pressure and overload, Dr. Clown has succeeded in impacting the medical-care team as well, and changing the atmosphere.

We are writing this letter with a heartfelt plea, but along with this we would not wish to hide our amazement and anger at this unfortunate step. It is difficult to understand this situation both on the financial level (this will, after all, be a minor saving) as well as on the value level which is incompatible with all of the hospital's declarations and of the mission statement of care, the importance of the mental and emotional well-being of the patients and their families.

Please, we beg of you—do not take Dr. Clown away from us. You should not have science and pure medicine alone suffice. Remember the function of the mind in healing the body, and enable us, in the midst of our suffering, to have a smile and a deep breath.

Sincerely,

[names omitted]

cc: Director General, Medical Center, Central Israel
Director General of the Hospital
Director of the network of Oncology Departments
Deputy Director of the network of Oncology Departments
Deputy Director of the Hospital
Director, Cancer Center
Director, Oncology Day Care Unit, Oncology Department
Assistant to the Director General of the Hospital, central Israel
Director, Center for Supportive Medicine

Director of the Division of Media, Publicity and
    Strategic Marketing
Executive Director of the Israel Cancer Association
Spokesperson, Director of the Informational Depart-
    ment, Israel Cancer Association
Executive Director, Philnor Foundation-The Dream
    Doctors Project

The director of the oncology day-care unit also sent a courageous
letter to the hospital administration, noting the fact that many of
the patients did indeed schedule their appointments for treatment
according to the clown doctor's work days. She did not stop there,
but went on to state that in cutting-edge, technology-based medicine, emotion-based aspects are often neglected—medical clowning
at least provides a partial response to this need. Finally, she criti-
cized the termination notice, and objects to the hospital's declarations. Following is a translation of the letter [all names have been
deleted here as well]:

> **To:** The Director of the Research Fund, Medical Center,
> central Israel
>
> Dear Sir,
>
> > **Re:** Request to Cancel the Termination of Employ-
> > ment of Dr. Clown—Medical Clown, Oncology
> > Day Clinic
>
> I am writing this letter to ask you to cancel the decision to
> terminate Mr. Dr. Clown's employment at the hospital's
> oncology day clinic. Dr. Clown has been working there for
> the past two years. Although a certain skepticism accom-
> panied him initially—"A medical clown? On an adult
> ward?"—after a few of his sessions, he became an integral
> and appreciated part of the medical-care team at the day
> clinic, where both patients and staff eagerly awaited his
> arrival. The cynicism melted away as if it had never been.

It's no secret that most "healthy" people prefer not to set foot in a place like the day clinic, preferring not to think about it, or not to fear it for it won't happen to them. But, au contraire, Dr. Clown entered the clinic with confidence, bringing with him joie de vivre and a promise of health. In a creative way, using his ingenious skills, the Doc knows how to bond with patients, instill calm, and elicit responses—from smiles to hearty laughs—but, mainly, to make people forget for a few moments, or, at least, to paint with brighter colors the dark picture of the daily reality which the patients endure. He is skilled at giving the medical-care staff the space they need so as not to disturb their work; at the same time, he makes it easier for the patients to receive the treatment. This is a fact, because there are patients who ask especially to schedule their appointments on the days that which Dr. Clown will be at work. Further proof of this lies in the fact that a letter was written and signed by dozens of patients, testifying to Dr. Clown's unique contribution to their lives.

The Oncology Institute and the Medical Center have recently publicized their "mission statement," that is, to provide holistic care for the oncology patient, treatment that envelopes the patient and responds to all aspects of the illness, including emotional and mental needs which often tend to be neglected by the technology- and innovation-driven system.

Taking all this into consideration, the decision to make the budget cut exactly here, axing the valuable human resource providing even a most partial response to this vision, is all the more surprising, and contradicts, in practice, all of the recent notifications and advertisements issued by the Hospital in its approach.

I hereby invite all those associated with this issue to arrive in person to the oncology day clinic, to form your own impressions of Dr. Clown's work. And I am asking you to once again weigh this matter, taking serious consideration of the issue, and enable him to continue his work in the day clinic.

Sincerely,

Director, Oncology Day Clinic, The Oncology Institute, Medical Center, Central Israel

The administration's response to the letters was immediate—and negative. Due to budget cuts, we are forced to terminate the medical clown's employment. This reaction angered the patients, especially after, that same week, the financial newspaper *Calcalist* (April 10, 2014) ran a report on the outrageously high salaries of senior hospital officials. The patients decided to continue their fight to have Dr. Clown continue at the Medical Center, and turned to the media. On Friday, April 11, popular Israeli daily *Yedioth Ahronoth* wrote about the patients versus the administration, and the article was posted on the newspaper's Facebook page. Thousands of "likes" and dozens of comments followed. Some examples of the emotional responses follow:

> Under no circumstances in any way should you make any cuts in the services provided by the medical clown. I know Dr. Clown personally. He is an amazing person performing extremely important work of making patients smile. The saying, "Laughter is the best medicine" is no empty statement. Dr. Clown, you precious person, we are with you!!!

> Hey everybody, share share share!!!!!! I am a cancer patient, and I know this fantastic person who brings smiles to people's faces. I was hospitalized this week and was so happy to see Dr. Clown, do me a favor and forward this, it's a crying shame to stop the patients' bright spot.

> Dr. Clown saves lives!

It's all for the best . . . everything's temporary . . . only good will come of this . . . Dr. Clown's job is of inestimable value.

That cute Dr. Clown makes everyone laugh. He contributes a great deal to the patients, encourages them and makes them smile. Do not make the budget cuts on him!!!!! I know how important he is to the patients there!!!

He is a wonderful person who is doing extremely important work . . . My dear mother has been in the oncology ward for many weeks, and each time he comes to the ward, she has a smile and an expression of happiness! We will do our utmost to keep Dr. Clown with us . . . Happy holiday, and may you have good health.

It's a crying shame what an unfortunate decision by the person in charge of financing the medical clown for a ward like this one, instead of adding more work hours to the medical clown, they think they should remove him. Let the hospital director with a high salary or the other department directors let them have their salaries cut to finance the hours on behalf of the cancer patients. To hell with it what's happening here in our country, how low can we go.

The newspaper also published the hospital administration's response:

> The service provided by the medical clowns is important, but clearly, under the present budgetary pressure, this type of service has to be sacrificed. Despite the aforesaid, the administration of the medical center will do everything to seek donors who can help.

Their statement did not satisfy the patients, because they wondered how it was possible for the hospital to fail to find a budgetary allocation for one medical clown, that too for only eight hours a week even though the medical clowning was so vital to their facility. The patients felt that it was an especially "low blow" because of the high salaries of the hospital administrators, far exceeding the salary levels for top civil servants in the country. Although people with cancer usually do not have energy to spare—surely not for those undergoing chemotherapy—they decided to continue their protest through the media, and ensure the clown doctor remained on his job. The patients contacted the media again, and in the online version of the national newspaper, put forth the plea to cancel the decision to terminate the medical clown's employment.

After repeated letters and exchanges with the media, Dr. Clown was informed that he could, in the meantime, continue to work in the hospital's oncology units.

This was a foundational narrative in the medical clown's professional life. The patients' intense emotions, especially when expressing how meaningful the clown's work in the hospital was for them, was an extremely moving experience for the medical clown . . .

CHAPTER TEN

Clowning with the "Enemy"
Medical Clowning in Natural Disasters and Conflict Zones

For medical clowns, crises arising from violent conflicts or natural disasters provide the opportunity to bring the memory of positive emotions and joie de vivre to the community through their unique performative abilities. The medical clowns mediate the humor and imagination for the community suffering from extensive trauma due to a natural disaster or war, in the same way in which they use humor and imagination to mediate for patients undergoing personal trauma due to illness or painful treatment procedures. The medical clowns thus facilitate the beginning of a process of healing and rehabilitation on both the individual and community levels.

In January 2010, several days after an earthquake struck Haiti, three medical clowns arrived in Port au Prince, as part of the mission of the Israeli Flying Aid (IFA), a non-profit organization which extends humanitarian assistance. The three "Dream Doctors," Hamutal Ende, Shuli Victor, and Dudi Barashi, who work as medical clowns in hospitals in Israel as part of the Dream Doctors Project, joined the mission to help the wounded in the field hospital (set up by the Israel Defense Forces), in orphanages, and outside among the debris.

Medical clowning uses a concept called "entering the room," referring to the way in which the medical clown comes into the patient's room. In Haiti, Dudi Barashi called this "entering the abyss." In a talk at the University of Haifa,[1] Dudi and Hamutal described the audience before whom they appeared—a community greatly traumatized, both physically and emotionally. The work was intensive, lasting many hours, including one-on-one work with the wounded in the field hospital, with orphans in children's homes run by the missionary, and an out-of-doors clowning performance for hundreds of onlookers. While work in the field hospital was more like the medical clowns' regular jobs, the work outside was more similar to street theater, only this time it was for an audience who had lost their near and dear ones as well as all their homes and everything else they possessed. The audience was traumatized and in social chaos; they had no vital services either, for the state had totally collapsed in the earthquake.

Prof. Mooli Lahad, president of Community Stress Prevention in Israel, has said that in disaster zones such as Haiti, the medical clowns are able to create an "island of resilience" where laughter and playfulness take place. They create an interactive zone of activities, and in this sense, they facilitate a "sense of community" which helps people begin the long process of recovery.[2]

Dr. Susana Pendzik, of the Hebrew University of Jerusalem, while speaking of medical clowns' activities in disaster zones, says that the clown, as an archetype, represents universal imagination and activates fantasy in people suffering from PTSD, thus stimulating their inborn capacity to cope with crisis.

In December 2004, a group of Dream Doctors medical clowns joined a humanitarian mission to Thailand following the devastating tsunami. Nimrod Eisenberg, one of the medical clowns, described how the games they initiated (in which survivors were active participants) helped everyone address their loss and suffering. Another Dream Doctor, Yaron Goshen, described one of the games where a group of children acted out the tsunami while another group fled from it so as not to be caught. He stated that the game provided an emotional release, and allowed the fleeing children to curse and scream at the "Tsunami."

Prof. Lahad has also stated that medical clowning is effective and capable of positively impacting the communities which have experienced catastrophe and trauma.[3]

Another organization specializing in performing in disaster zones is Clowns Without Borders. Established in Barcelona in July

1993 by Tortell Poltrona, it started with performances for children in a refugee camp in Croatia during the civil war which followed the separation of Yugoslavia. The organization went on to found branches in Belgium, Canada, France, Germany, Ireland, South Africa, Spain, and the United States. Over the past decade, Clowns Without Borders have performed for trauma victims in disaster zones throughout the world, and helped people and comunities cope with the aftermath of natural disasters and armed conflicts.

There are three types of clowning performances in trauma zones:

a. The first is the medical clown's performance in makeshift field hospitals in the disaster zone, usually set up by aid missions coming in from outside the country (for example, in Haiti). The foreign humanitarian missions step into the vacuum created by the collapse of the healthcare systems, a situation made worse by the scarcity of basic medicine or even clean drinking water, etc. Medical clowning in a field hospital is not essentially different from the routine practice in hospitals, except for the unusual intensity of the trauma and the pace of the work. The medical clown often works individually with one-on-one interactions with the patient based on improvisation and gags suited to the personality of the patient.

b. The second type of clowning is the street-theater clowning or circus clowning, in a carefully orchestrated performance (usually a group show) of comic-circus skills in front of an audience in a makeshift arena. The interaction with the audience is not personal—it is a response to the need for a restorative experience for a community reeling from a traumatic experience. The performance attempts to fulfill the need for a holistic therapy. Although rooted in the traumatic reality, it creates an alternative reality in order to ease the pain and suffering and to maked it possible for the community to express and share its stories.

c. The third type of clowning is the activity performance, similar to a birthday-party clowning or day-camp clowning, in which the audience actively participates in amusing tasks performed by the clown. These joint activities, in which the audience carries out the funny "assignments", have effective therapeutic qualities for the individual as well as the community recovering from the trauma of some kind of natural or man-made disaster.

Medical clowning facilitates the human connection, and makes it possible for people on both sides of the conflict to express mutual understanding, brotherhood, and objection to their position as people trapped in a sitation forced upon them. Moreover, it is detrimental for either side—a conflict disrupts lives for ever and extracts a steep price.

The Barzilai Medical Center in Ashqelon, where I worked as a medical clown, is at the front, located about 10 kilometers from Gaza, as the crow flies. Since 2004, I worked at the hospital with patients suffering from PSTD and injuries, most of them from the Israeli villages near the border, but also from Gaza.

The hospital was also a target for the rockets launched from Gaza. Luckily, none damaged the unshielded hospital structure. At the time, Barzilai Medical Center was a separate emotional territory: outside of its walls the chaotic and violent reality of war (with vicious "rounds" being fired over the years, with the most violent barrages in late 2008 and early 2009). In an absurd scene, the Jews and Arabs on the medical staff were treating Jews and Arabs wounded in a war arising from the religious and national differences between Jews and Arabs.

This was truly "the hour of the medical clown."

Because the medical clowns have no national or religious identity, the clown doctor can "skip over" such cultural markers. The clown is a universal archetype, representing imagination and humor in all cultures, without belonging to any one; therein lies the power of clowning. The clown can bring together people from opposing sides into an imaginary, humorous extraterritorial uni-verse, an alternative reality, to counter their relentless struggle for survival in the conflict zone. Although each clown has a real person behind the persona—someone with a cultural identity and socio-political tendencies—he or she identifies with the patients on a human level. Clowns who become the mouthpiece of political propaganda of any kind or those who allow political or cultural identities to slip into their work are making a serious error in their professional career.

Medical clowning enabled me to create a bridge between chil-dren and adults from both sides of the conflict—the encounters that provided inspiration and hope for me, especially for our diffi-cult region of the Middle East. I would like to describe several of these encounters here.

While working as a medical clown in one of the orthopedic wards at Barzilai Medical Center, I met Yossi, a 10-year-old Israeli boy, wounded in the shoulder by a Qassam rocket that was launched from Gaza on his town of Sderot. Wounded by shrapnel, the boy managed to seek shelter in a small supermarket where a TV crew was also sheltering while it documented the minutes fol-lowing the attack and Yossi's medical evacuation. In the next room was Jihad, a Palestinian boy from Gaza, wounded by Israeli attacks. Near Jihad were Israeli children. Khaled, a young boy from Gaza, used to run down the corridor of the pediatrics unit together with Daniel, a Jewish–Israeli boy from Ashkelon, screaming with joy every time I "almost stumbled" as I fled from them with clownish clumsiness.

The hospital rooms, with the Israeli and Palestinian child patients together, all wounded physically and suffering from seri-ous mental trauma, transformed into the sites of big parties when I arrived, the children and their families wiggling in wild dances to the rhythm of my drumming on the guitar, as if there were no war outside. The rhythm made everyone move, and the clown "farts" (from my "fart machine") made them all laugh. Yossi and

Ahmad were surprised, then burst into peals of laughter when I explained in gibberish—and mimicked with outrageous hand movements—how to take care of stomach pains while operating my "fart machine" from the back pocket of my trousers.

Professional literature makes no mention of medical clowning during wartime, nor describes any healing performances in a hospital caring for children from the warring sides, those who have been injured and wounded in the vicious nexus of attacks–counterattacks. As a medical clown, I had the feeling of being in a theatre of the absurd, in which the arena of the hospital was an island of sanity. No less surreal were my feelings during interviews by TV crews in which I attempted to describe the experiences of the wounded children from the medical clown's perspective.[4]

Beyond Country Borders and Beyond the Limits of My Inner Clown

This story takes place (and is still taking place at the time of writing) in the pediatrics unit at Chaim Sheba Medical Center. It is the story of a friendship formed over many years during which I crossed the frontiers of my clown persona. As a leading medical center located in central Israel, dozens of Palestinian children arrive in the ward each month for various complex treatments. In 2010, in the North B unit, I first met young Mochi and his grandfather Hamouda from Khan Yunis in the southern Gaza Strip. Mochi was only a few months old, suffering from an extremely rare intestinal infection—just over a few dozen similar cases have been diagnosed in the world. There was no care for his disease in Gaza, so they had come to Israel for treatment.

Grandpa Hamouda volunteered to accompany the baby because neither his mother nor his father were able to, nor wanted to, come to Israel with little Mochi. When I first met them as a medical clown, I had no idea that this would be a friendship that would last many long years. I encountered a baby who was always cheerful, despite the pain that had become an inseparable part of his life. He was very interested in the colorful soap bubbles I blew for him, in the sounds I made, the taps and notes emanating from my guitar and harmonica, the various items and little dolls that sprouted from my bag of tricks and came to life. Grandpa Hamouda, a very impressive man, with a thick white beard and piercing blue eyes, was always very happy to see me, and would notify his grandbaby in a very festive tone that I was on my way the second he spotted me at the end of the corridor. Later, he joined me in the clowning for his grandson.

The days turned into weeks, and the weeks stretched into months: Grandpa Hamouda realized that they would not be returning to to his wife and children in Khan Yunis, because Baby Mochi's condition was not yet stable. Since the beginning of our acquaintance, I was very impressed by Hamouda's devotion to his grandson. Mochi did not know his parents; in fact, he knew no other world except that of the hospital. Hamouda informally adopted his grandson and became his sole guardian. "Besides being a grandfather, I'm his mother as well as his father," he used to say, never leaving the baby's side. We developed a close friendship—Hamouda and I—as well as a deep affection for little Mochi. Each time I visited them, we would dance and sing to the baby while he would rock in the crib, holding the side rail with one hand and drumming on them with the other. As I met with them over the years, I ventured beyond the limits of my professional medical clown persona. I was no longer just the medical clown but Amnon, the private citizen. The encounter with Hamouda was an opportunity, almost impossible outside of the hospital space—for two people on the opposing sides of a difficult national conflict to bond as two human beings, untouched by the conflict raging between our people for more than a century.

About a year before we met, a difficult war was taking place between Israel and Gaza. From December 27, 2008 to January 18, 2009, hundreds of rockets were launched form Gaza toward civilian targets, many landing near my house in Ashkelon. Several fell on my street, and damaged my neighbors' homes. Hamouda had worse luck: an Israeli counterattack destroyed his home and the sheepfold, his main source of income. Luckily, his family was unhurt, and they moved in with his father. Now he was on a long list of those awaiting aid from UNRWA to rebuild his house. We both felt a great sense of hope in our meeting and our clowning performances for Mochi. It was our joint personal therapy, liberating us from the suspicion and hostility enveloping us all like the strands of a giant spider web.

Young Mochi needed a blood-marrow donation as well as a large financial donation. Because the Palestinian Authority and Hamas were unwilling to pay for any more treatments, I approached a friend who had contacts in the media. Within a few hours the local news-channel crew arrived to film Mochi and Hamouda for a breaking-news feature that very day, hoping to find a donor. Several people phoned after the TV spot, but no donor was found.

Mochi loved to dance to the rhythm of the guitar; he moved his body and mimicked the music, because he understood both Hebrew and Arabic, and was loved by the staff.

Unfortunately, because of Mochi's weak immune system, he was infected with a vicious strain of bacteria and was admitted to the intensive care unit. His condition was critical—he had to be intubated and ventilated. Hamouda broke down and told me that Mochi was on his way to . . . and pointed to the heavens. Our little Mochi lingered between heaven and earth for 10 days in the ICU, on the ventilator, with tubes attached to him, his little body entirely darkened. I stood near him and sang quietly—all of the songs he loved—hoping that he would hear something. Ten days later, Mochi began to show signs of emerging out of it. He regained a healthy complexion but only till his torso; his limbs remained dark, for gangrene had developed in all four limbs, leaving the doctors no choice but to amputate them in order to save his life.

For weeks after the amputations, Mochi was in a most depressed state, gloomy and withdrawn, and obviously in a great deal of pain. He would look at me, but hardly react to my clowning. He would try to take something from me or strum my guitar then remember he had no hands, and then he would look at his stumps and sigh. When the pain reduced a bit, we developed the "Dance of the Eyebrows" together. Instead of dancing, he moved his eyebrows to the rhythm of my guitar and harmonica. He accompanied the movement with funny mimicry and a huge smile, making everyone around him laugh. At that time, he had very painful treatment procedures; even putting cream on his stumps and taking blood from his neck caused him great pain. I actively took part in the procedures, trying to make him laugh to divert his attention, and he tried his best to play along. Sometimes he would sing with me, and at other times he would do the "eyebrow dance" with a tearful smile until the pain became too much for him and he would shriek, alternating with smiles, all during the procedures. It took weeks, but gradually he began to heal.

By then, Mochi was now almost 3 years old.

One day I suggested to Hamouda that we go for a trip to the zoo and safari park in the nearby city. It is difficult to describe the tremendous impact this trip had on Mochi. He was outside the hospital for the first time since coming there as an infant and, of course, he had no memory of life before the hospital. When we got into my car, he was amazed. At the zoo, he was gloriously happy to see all of the animals. Some of the time, we pushed him in a carriage, some of the time he asked me to carry him. Imitating the animal noises and mimicking their expressions later became an integral part of our clowning interaction.

After Mochi recovered from the surgeries, and his disease seemed to become more dormant, Hamouda decided to return to their home in the Gaza.

But during the 10 days they were in Khan Yunis, Mochi's condition deteriorated; he began to run a high fever and sores broke out all over his body. Mochi's father, who had not seen him since

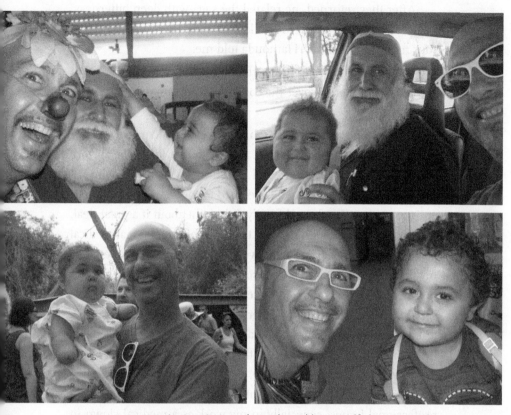

FIGURE 10.1 (TOP LEFT). Amnon Raviv with Mochi and his grandfather Hamouda at Chaim Sheba Medical Center, Tel HaShomer, 2010. FIGURE 10.2 (TOP RIGHT). On the way to the zoo, Ramat Gan, 2013. FIGURE 10.3 (BOTTOM LEFT). With Mochi at the safari park, Ramat Gan, 2013. FIGURE 10.4 (BOTTOM RIGHT). With young Mochi at the Chaim Sheba Medical Center, 2014.

he left for the hospital as a baby, came to see him, spent 10 minutes with him and rejected him. Hamouda told me that Mochi's father suggested abandoning him near a mosque where Fate could decide what would happen to him. The mother said that he had no place in their family; his younger siblings punched him as the poor kid lay there, helpless. Hamouda decided he would return to the hospital, but the Hamas authorities would not allow him to leave unless he signed a document stating he would never ask for money for treatments for Mochi in an Israeli hospital.

After they returned, he related the saga with deep bitterness. "When we were in Gaza, Mochi kept mentioning you, and called your name all the time," Hamouda told me.

Back in the hospital, the staff stabilized the child's condition and found a donor to cover the costs of his treatment and rehabilitation.

At the same time, my daughter was hospitalized for a short time in the same pediatrics ward. She, of course, knew the doctors and nurses as well as Mochi and the other children with whom I worked. Every aspect of my life seemed to merge—clowning, parenting, concern, work, and family. I thought about it a great deal, wondering about borderlines and the limits of professional medical clowning. Did they exist? What were the desirable limits between my professional life and my personal life? Apparently, the answer to this question is a personal one, and each medical clown must set his own limits according to personality and specific cases. Medical clowns are committed to breaking all borders and consensus, including the rules they set for themselves. After all, this is the essence of clowning. In any case, I challenge my limits as a practicing professional, and constantly introspect on the personal–professional issues, especially in my work as a medical clown in adult wards with patients with life-threatening and terminal illnesses.

Young Mochi was transferred to the Rehabilitation Department where he was fitted with small-sized prosthetic limbs. He practiced walking, eating, and carrying out all kinds of tasks. Although I had been transferred to the adult oncology wards, I would visit him at the end of the day, still in my clown attire, to give an exclusive performance for Mochi and his friends. I usually performed in the small lunchroom of the department, along with all of the other children and their parents. We would hold a "grand feast" accompanied by singing and dancing. Mochi seemed to be full of energy; he was joyous again. He ate with good appetite, and learnt to ride a tricycle, pedaling rapidly with his prostheses. Every few months, his grandmother, Hamouda's wife, would come for a visit, and Mochi would chatter and sing to her in Hebrew and Arabic.

Hamouda traveled to Gaza a few times for family events. Each time he had to undergo exhausting an interrogation process by the Hamas Police. When he returned the last time, he made the final decision that since Mochi had no future in Gaza, and would not survive there, he would request a permanent residency for himself and his grandson in Israel. With the assistance of Israeli friends, their story was publicized in the Israeli media.

At the time of writing, Mochi is still in the Rehabilitation Department, practicing everyday tasks using his prostheses. He is now 6 and half years old. Grandpa Hamouda is by his side as he has been for all these years. I still come in as a medical clown, but mainly as a friend, to dance the "eyebrow dance" with Mochi, to laugh, sing, and talk with Hamouda about life. We talk about how things could have been without all the needless wars which have made our lives miserable.

Over the last few months, I have been coming to the lunch-room at Rehabilitation Department. After Mochi and Hamouda finish eating, we sing Hebrew and Arabic songs. Mochi may be the only toddler who has been raised on children's songs in languages of both of the sides involved in this unceasing conflict.

Notes

1   In October 2010, University of Haifa organized the event "I was in Haiti," where volunteers and representatives of relief and res-cue operations where invited. The event presented a documen-tary on the work of medical clowns associated with Dream Doctors Project, and their relentless effort to light up the dark-ness shrouding Haiti after the devastating earthquake. For a video of the talk by Dudi Barashi and Hamutal Ende I refer to here, please see "I Was in Haiti," University of Haifa YouTube Channel (October 13, 2010). Available in Hebrew at: https://-goo.gl/cRg9z7 (last accessed on July 1, 2017).

2 For a video on the Dream Doctors working in Haiti earthquake, the Tsunami in Thailand, Indonesia earthquake, and the Middle East conflict zone, please see "Inside the Trauma Zone," Dream Doctors Israel Archives (November 14, 2010). Available at: https://goo.gl/MtTJ7b (last accessed on July 1, 2017).

3 In August 2010, a workshop was held in Ami'ad to train Dream Doctors to perform in situations of adversity and disaster, such as war, natural disasters, and paricipate in humanitarian missions aiding the various public service organizations. For a short documentary feature this workshop, see "A Refort On the Preparatory Workshop," Dream Doctors Israël Archives(August 24, 2010). Available at: https://goo.gl/01wgcH (last accessed on July 3, 2017).

4 The video footage of this interview on Channel 2, Israeli TV, is accessible on the author's YouTube Channel. See "Interview with Amnon Raviv: Medical Clown during Operation Cast Lead," ARaviv (June 2, 2010). Available at: https://goo.gl/NBTwn3 (last accessed on July 3, 2017).

CHAPTER ELEVEN

Save the Clown!

The Clown Doctor and Compassion Fatigue

Medical clowning is not an easy profession emotionally, especially when the medical clown works on palliative care wards or with patients suffering from serious and life-threatening illnesses. In these departments, the clowns are exposed to the patients' and their families' deep pain and anxiety, a burden which is not easy to bear. It affects the clowns on a cumulative basis, and, like other medical professionals and paraprofessionals, medical clowns are likely to develop compassion fatigue whose symptoms are very similar to trauma reactions.

In "Compassion Fatigue and Burnout," J. Benson and K. Magraith have argued that a psychologist-led support group for those at risk of developing compassion fatigue due to their professional work with the seriously ill has been shown to be efficacious in lessening that risk (2005). In addition to participation in a care group, personal calming and humorous activities have a beneficial effect.

John Luquette has said that a range of individual actions can help nurses working in oncology departments—for example, proposing guided imagery, setting boundaries, meditation, muscle relaxation exercises, and supportive group activities (2007).

Similarly, medical clowns working in certain departments and witnessing agonizing pain and suffering every day are at risk of burnout and compassion fatigue, perhaps even more than physicians and nurses. The essential element of the medical clown's work is based on their personal bonding and significant interaction with patients while the medical personnel's work is not measured by parameters of mutual enjoyment but, rather, by the carrying out medical procedures.

Indices for the medical clowns' professional work evaluate the pleasure and the human connection which facilitates the expression of humor and imagination that clowns and patients share. Studies recommend the organization of professional support groups, balanced personal and professional lives, and relaxation activities aimed at reducing the risk of compassion fatigue among members of the staff.

There is an additional and important factor moderating compassion fatigue and burnout—the satisfaction felt by the medical staff. The more the caregiver on the medical team cares for the self, using techniques of support groups and personal attention, the lower the feeling of compassion fatigue or burnout, and the greater the feeling of compassion satisfaction (Alkema, Linton, and Davies 2008).

In interviews I conducted with 20 medical clowns from the Dream Doctors Project, some reported compassion fatigue after years of working in oncology departments, hospice care, intensive care, and other wards. Some reported very painful emotions after a child, whom they had accompanied through long periods of hospitalization, passed away. With some, it was expressed in periodic energy "lows," lack of desire to go to work, and burnout. One medical clown described the feeling in picturesque terms: "You have to understand that a medical clown is a person who 'burns bright,' because if he's not working 'full steam ahead,' he's not doing the job." That medical clown realized that he had to find a balance, and told me that one of the things that helps him to emotionally cope is to sit down at the end of the workday and reconstruct in his mind what he has gone through that day.

All of the respondents reported compassion satisfaction, a feeling that the work was very rewarding, and that they were being repaid with great gratitude from patients and staff, all of which helped with their emotional coping. All medical clowns spoke of the sharing with other Dream Doctors or colleagues (in groups or personal conversations) their inner struggles or distress due to the work, as one of the ways to address the difficulties.

When a medical clown accompanying a patient, battling an illness over months and even years, sees them recuperate, it is an empowering experience. As one medical clown related to me, "I succeeded in undergoing an entire experience from the beginning, through the middle to the end, and I had the privilege of seeing the change though my very eyes. This gave me a tremendous amount of strength, knowing that I took part in the child's recovery."

The clowns also explained how the work impacts their personal lives. One medical clown told me that it took him time to understand and associate the instances in which his outbursts of rage at his wife and children was in many ways related to the difficult experiences he was having in the hospital.

But there is also a reverse effect, from home to hospital, as described by a woman clown: "If I come to work after some unpleasantness at home, then I'm not as strong as I should be on the job, and it affects me more quickly . . . I definitely feel the burnout after many years of working . . . I don't know how long I will continue."

The number of years working as a medical clown is, of course, significant, on the one hand for the feeling of emotional burden of care, and on the other for the necessity of developing a "shock absorber," a mechanism preventing burnout at work. Another clown described it thus: "Nowadays, I won't come to work exposed. I used to come without any 'filters,' but now I have my filters. I don't need to seal myself behind a big wall, but I do have a 'transparent bubble' around me . . . At first, every little thing pierced my heart, flooded me to the extent that I couldn't contain it any more. I used to cry easily, then I would go home with all of the stories and didn't know how to cope, I would be flooded with emotions and didn't know what do to with all of those feelings and deep emotions."

The Philnor Foundation set up a group-support mechanism so that the medical clowns could cope with their problems. Group meetings were held over the years, facilitated by professionals and providing case-by-case responses to the stories published in a closed online forum.

Clinical psychologist Prof. Gil Goldzweig, from the Academic College of Tel Aviv-Yaffo, provided professional support to the medical clowns working under the Dream Doctors Project during the first few years of operation. I asked him in an interview in April 2014 about the issues that distressed the medical clowns and the most frequent subjects brought up in the forum. Prof. Goldzweig emphasized that he had accompanied the Project from its inception, and that some of the initial issues with which the medical clowns were struggling were associated with their professional identity. Questions of meaning arose, such as, "Is what we are doing really helping anyone?" He noted the similarity to questions arising in support groups of medical staff members, although in a weaker formulation. During the first few years of the Project, the lack of professional self-confidence was evident, which gave rise to issues of borders, such as: how to relate to child patients when they became aggressive toward the medical clown; or if the medical clown should stop playacting while interacting with the medical staff because it was necessary to discuss a case. How close should the clown get to a patient and their family? Should the medical clown attend the funeral of a child patient to whom they had grown close?

Another issue was the medical clown's isolated position. Most of the Dream Doctors worked alone, and had no other clowns to whom they could ask their questions: How were they to deal with the emotional overload from the suffering and death they witnessed at work? And what about the cumulative feeling of inner distress: How should they deal with this when coming home to their families? I asked Prof. Goldzweig whether there were unique traits in the medical clown's personality which make it easier or

more difficult to cope with what happens in the hospital, as compared with the medical-care staff. He explained that medical clowns
have more issues of existential identity. In general, the medical
clowns ask themselves, "Who am I, and what am I?" They look
both inward and outward. Whereas he came up against much
fewer questions such as these from physicians and nurses.

When I asked him whether medical clowns "become immune"
to traumatic experiences of pain and death, since they are often
exposed to this in their work with child patients, he argued that
studies have shown there is no such "immunization;" medical
clowns sometimes become apathetic but that is only a symptom.
He recommends that beginners start working in the units where
the child patients are not suffering from very serious illnesses, and
only those with substantial experience should practice in the more
difficult departments. He noted that a built-in part of the medical
clown's work is to challenge boundaries, as long as these are
boundaries "behind the red nose." Behind the figure of the medical
clown is a "safe area," but when a case tests the borderline between
the clown persona and the clown as human being, Goldzweig
states that there lies the danger of "destabilization."

Dr. Shlomit Bresler was the facilitator of the Dream Doctors'
support group from 2010 to 2012. They met once a month—too
infrequently, according to Dr. Bresler—with the goal of enabling
the medical clowns to share and discuss their emotional experiences, to bring up distressing issues and troubling questions and
seek support from the group. Dr. Bresler remembers that a significant issue that appeared in these meetings was the difficulty in
dealing with the death of a child patient with whom a clown had
worked. This was such a painful issue, and impossible to contain.
One of the clowns said that when she eventually went to heaven,
she would meet groups of children there. Meeting with the children
and the families, the human identification and the tragedy of the
death of a child, is a trauma for the medical clown. The questions
that arose were not only about how to deal with the death but, often,

about how to respond to the parents' request to attend the funeral and the mourning period in their home, about how much involvement is acceptable, and about how close they should be to the family, that is, about whether they should visit them outside the hospital.

What is the place of the medical clown in the healthcare team? This was another pressing issue that arose. Is the medical clown part of the staff? What is the medical clown's professional identity, and what is a medical clown? What exactly is their role? These are questions which do not involve death and secondary traumatization, but, nevertheless, over time, do impact medical clowns' compassion fatigue.

I asked Dr. Bresler if she could point to differences between how beginners and "old-timers" dealt with such questions, especially those regarding death. She described the significant differences in the level of professional confidence: the experienced medical clowns shared their insights with the beginners and described how, over time, they developed existential tools to cope with death, although death shook them up no less deeply despite their years on the job. Dr. Bresler did not describe their attitude as a lack of emotion or imperviousness; rather, the experienced medical clowns had a different sense of understanding and tolerance formed over their years of work.

Medical clowns who had young children at home had a higher level of anxiety than those who were not parents. This was due to their greater identification and fear that the illnesses and death might, Heaven forbid, strike their own children too.

Medical clowns who worked with adults wondered about how to adapt their clowning for adults, and about how close should they become to their patients. Medical clowns participating in painful medical procedures, such as in the burn unit, found it difficult to contain such an intense level of pain among the patients over such a long time. Personal temperament was another issue: What happens if the medical clown has to be at work and "is not in the mood?" This is very troubling for the beginners while those who have been working for a long time think that the medical clown must always be authentic and spontaneous. If the medical clown is feeling "low," the best thing to do is to channel the mood into comedy.

When I asked Dr. Bresler about the desirable personality traits in medical clowns which might help address their compassion fatigue, she said, "Medical clowns are very intelligent people, and, of course, they have a very well-developed sense of humor." She noted that even when the meetings touched upon sensitive subjects, they were full of good humor and laughter. The sense of belonging to a group, and having the opportunity to share and hear others, empowers them to cope with the challenging aspects of their work. Dr. Bresler concluded by stating that the strength of the group lay in the sharing with each other rather than in finding a solution to professional or ethical dilemmas. These are extremely personal issues and there are no straightforward answers.

Prof. Rachel Lev-Wiesel, head of the Graduate School of Creative Art Therapies, University of Haifa, told me in an interview in April 2014, of her hypothesis that medical clowns are in need of dissociative characteristics, a certain emotional alienation from the painful situations they witness. The biochemical mechanism of this severance takes place in the brain, as the mirror neurons resonate with others' experiences to facilitate empathy for their sufferings. Prof. Lev-Wiesel stated that medical clowns develop a very mild dissociative disorder that enables them to shift their state of ego, in the same way that some of the greatest actors consciously practice. The actor "is located" in a different time and space, and the greatness of their craft lies in the ability to transport the audience into that time and space, into that fictive reality. The medical clown, too, is "located" in a different place, a place which does not exist within the hospital, and he or she tries to "sweep the patient away" to that other realm. The big difference is that while the actor tries to transport the audience to the fictive realms created by the playwright, the medical clown tries to transport the patient suffering from pain and anxiety into the realms of humor and fantasy—a more physically and emotionally difficult task. In her opinion, this effort by the medical clown requires extremely high energy level which is one of the factors most likely to lead to compassion fatigue.

Another point which came up in our interview was the patient–medical clown relationship: a relationship not only develops between the patient and the clown persona but also with the individual beneath and behind the persona. Prof. Lev-Wiesel compared this to *Superman* in which Clark Kent is a "nobody" when he is not the Superman; he is just a "regular guy." The patients, like the audience, want their medical clown always in full possession of his or her unique powers. Because of this, and the euphoria at work, many medical clowns continue to remain "clowns" even when they are not on the job. This effort too leads to fatigue which in turn may cause depression. Perhaps this is the basis of a popular belief that clowns and comics are essentially sad people.

Based on my experiences, I can mention another element which did not come up in my interviews, nor did I find reference to it in any of the literature although it is definitely something that helps me deal with compassion fatigue—perhaps I can call it "compassion inspiration." I am referring to instances in which patients provide me with inspiration because of the way they coped with problems and challenges, and the strength they revealed under difficult, often impossible, conditions. These are situations which fill me with amazement and instill hope, for the human spirit—the soul—can cope with incredible challenges. I have witnessed cases that have changed my understanding of human nature, and my perspective of life, situations which have "recharged my batteries" at work as a medical clown and helped me address the emotional overload accumulated over a long period of time.

Some Recommendations

Medical clowning in the wards where patients are treated for serious diseases or in palliative care units is extremely challenging. It require tremendous inner strength to witness the suffering and death of patients whom the clown often accompanies for months and years. The medical clown's performance requires high mental and physical alertness, the ability to improvise and listen attentively, and the need to be available to the patient at all times. Due to intense involvement and routine practice, the clown may experience compassion fatigue and burnout. Other risk factors include lack of self-confidence in one's own clowning skills or because of the so-called inferior status within the hierarchy of the hospital system; isolation in the department (it is much easier for the medical clown when working in pairs or small groups); overlapping professional and personal lives; deep emotional involvement in the clown–patient interaction; and lack of innovation or professional training.

To mitigate the risk of developing compassion fatigue and burnout, we recommend the following to medical clowns:

a. Find your own path to achieve mental and physical balance and enhance your emotional quotient (pay attention to physical fitness, develop relaxation techniques, introspect, meditate, etc.). Try to strike a balance between your personal and professional lives—this will help you concentrate better and instill confidence, especially in the initial years of your career.

b. Join a support group which enables sharing and understanding between colleagues, preferably under the supervision of an experienced medical clown. (It can also be a closed online forum—but a professional facilitator is vital in this format as well.)

c. Find your personal "best match" to a specific department or a medical procedure. Understand what is most convenient for you; discuss with medical teams, and practice before you perform or assist in any procedure. Remember: not every medical clown is suited to work in every department.

d. If you are a beginner, we'd recommend that you start working with patients suffering from less severe ailments instead of attending to those who are terminally ill or undergoing more complex treatments. With experience and practice, you will be able to hone your skills and cope with greater professional challenges.

CHAPTER TWELVE

Humor in the "Twilight Zone"
My Work as a Medical Clown with Patients with Dementia

Nearly three decades have passed since the first program of medical clowning started in Babies and Children's Hospital of New York. While the vast majority of medical clowns still work with children in pediatric wards, over the past decade, more and more medical clowns have been working with adults and patients with dementia as part of holistic care. Medical clowning has unique advantages in working with patients with dementia, and several studies have shown that humor assists in improving the quality of life of such patients. The clown, as the ultimate comic figure, interacts with patients, engages them with simple activities, stimulates their cognitive abilities, and reinforces the patient's connection with their surroundings. In recent years, more clowns have been working with patients with dementia, most of them elderly, and with considerable success (Hendriks 2012).

Medical clowning with older patients with dementia differs from any other type of clowning because the disease affects the human consciousness. What does the patient with dementia feel, and how is it possible to negotiate the emotional aspects of the situation? Jacques and Jackson have stated that it is an error to think of a dementia patient as feeling imprisoned inside their own head without the capacities of memory or self-expression. It is incorrect to think of dementia as regression to a state of infancy, instead it is an experience of a fragmented world (2000). Patients fail to associate visions and sensations with meaning or significance. Jacques and Jackson claim that patients who are not seriously cognitively challenged can often express their feelings, as compared to those in a serious state of dementia who have no awareness of the environs or of their condition.

Taking the opposite view, Marion Violets states that the experience of a patient with dementia is indeed the feeling of being imprisoned inside one's own head, longing for the freedom which lies in clarity of thought (2000).

Perhaps both are correct, for different people must experience the illness differently, and the experience is individual and dependent on the patient's personality and severity of the illness.

Although the experience of dementia is not clear, its name clearly illustrates the way in which the society referred to those with the illness in the past. The source of the English word 'dementia' is from the Latin *de*, meaning without, outside of, or negation of *mens*, or the mind, that is, someone "out of their mind," or "mindless" person. The carnival clown has, similarly, been called "mindless" (Fiske 1989b).

Patients do not see the medical clown as a part of the hospital "system," nor consider the medical clown as a member of the staff. Consequently, they feel that the clown is their ally as opposed to the medical "establishment." This enables a unique interaction between the clown and older patients with dementia, which makes the patient feel better. They are also able to connect and engage with others, and the fact of having such a bond has a positive impact on their quality of life.

Many patients with dementia (especially in the early stages) understand that their condition will deteriorate in the future, and they strive to preserve their identity. Losing one's cognitive capacities causes fear, anxiety, disappointment, and lack of security. The interaction with the clown is free of any cognitive effort and improves the patient's feeling, since shared humor preserves the patient's sensation of the quality of life. The medical clown adapts himself to the patient's fragmented world; for clown and patient,

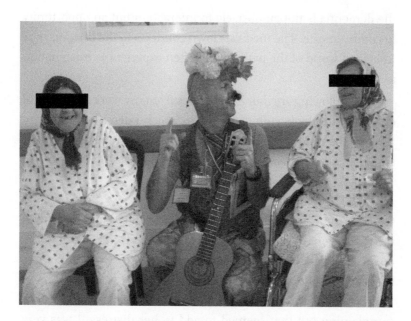

FIGURE 12.1 (ABOVE). A musical performance with patients with dementia. Harzfeld Hospital, Gedera, 2014.

FIGURE 12.2 (BELOW). Medical clown with a patient in dialysis care unit. Harzfeld Hospital, Gedera, 2014.

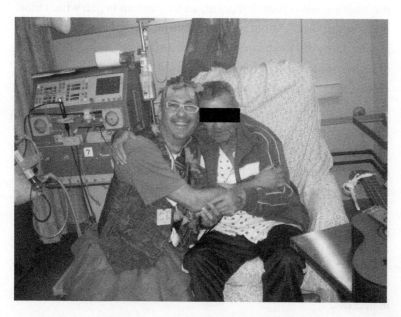

the dementia is not an obstacle to interaction but an opportunity to communicate. The medical clown connects to the imaginary or imagined world of the patient who often experiences imagination as reality.

The following are four case studies from my work as a medical clown with patients with dementia in which I describe the advantages of the unique clown–patient interaction in improving their spirits and their quality of life.*

The Line

One morning as I entered the ward at Hartzfeld Hospital, one of the older women patients named Dina was sitting in the lobby, crying because she had lost her number for the line. Of course, this had no connection with reality, since there was no queue in the ward except in her imagination. The nurses scolded her for complaining but that seemed to add to her distress. I was very interested and curious to know what the queue was for but her answer was unclear. I then drew the number "1" on a sheet of paper and gave it to her. Imemediately, Dina stopped crying and thanked me with a smile. From that point, an interaction began which took place in the "line". What we were waiting for was unclear, but the lack of clarity did not prevent the gift from being "realistic" for both of us. I invented a story full of improvised characters who then proceeded to converse with me and with Dina.

For patients with dementia, storytelling facilitates a release from "correct" or "incorrect" answers. The stories based on imagination and memory created with the patients are therapeutic, reflecting their longing for freedom and for acceptance from those around them. The characters who appear in Dina's story included her brother and his daughter who seldom visited her. Dina expressed her yearning for the relatives who appeared in her story whose plot moved between her need to wait in line for members

* All names of patients have been changed to protect the privacy of the individuals.

of the medical staff and her longing for her family. For Dina, the story facilitated the expression of emotions and provided an emotional release.

The Dance Party

Daphne, 85 years old, greets me with a big smile almost every time I visit their ward. Most of the time, she sits on her wheelchair in the lobby, speaking aloud—but it is hard to tell whether she is speaking to herself or to an elderly man sitting nearby. She tells me, "It's so good you arrived, because they're all here already." "Where is 'there'?" I ask her, ready and willing to jump into her imaginary world. It seems that the question surprises her, and she has to try very hard to remember. She scrabbles around in her memory, then says that they all went out dancing (although her response lacked confidence). "Of course," I reply, "but we must practice our waltz so that we'll be the best dancers at the party." I begin to waltz with Daphne while counting our steps out loud— "One, two, three, one, two, three." She looks at me with an amused look and says, "Lovely, very good." "Am I doing okay?" I ask her. "Yes, of course," she responds, "but let's go."

I take out my little tape recorder from my pocket and turn it on. The sounds of the *Libertango* by Astor Piazzolla fill the space of the lobby while in grotesque, over-exaggerated movements, I invite Daphne to dance with me. "All right," she says, and turns to the elderly man near her (engrossed in his own world), then looks at me as if unfolding a deep dark secret. "He's courting me," she says and stares into my eyes with a smile. I gently clutch her hand and grab the attached tray of the wheelchair with my other hand, and thus we dance in the lobby. I count out our steps, and draw the wheelchair after me according to the beat while Daphne laughs and hums the *Libertango*.

In the right kind of interaction, the medical clown seeks out a way to connect with the patient's world of feelings instead of bringing on a preconceived "work plan" to the encounter. One of the medical clown's advantages in working with patients is the varied range of artistic skills. The clown does not report to work as a therapist specializing in a specific discipline; they are not trained to employ a certain set of theories to any and all circumstances because the encounter with the patient will offer other possibilities. The clown is an interdisciplinary artist.

In this case, the subject of dance was brought up by the patient herself, and so it required a "clownish" response. Dancing with patients (even when the patient is in a wheelchair and her participation is restricted to hand movements) has a positive impact, and helps to calm the stormy emotions. Dance creates a positive arousal of the emotions among patients with dementia, with positive social significance. Daphne felt "courted" and expressed this when she interacted with other patients. The dance created a feeling of happiness and overall interest among the patients who looked on, and I went on to dance in the same way with everyone.

The Singer

Diana had been on the ward for several long months. Like Daphne, most of the time she was not exactly aware of where she was, and her blindness, coupled with her dementia, intensified her distress. Her usual place was in a wheelchair in the lobby. Sometimes she would stare quietly into space, but at most other times she would be crying, yelling, and calling for the nurse. When I sat down next to her, she would identify me by my voice, calm down and smile. And we had a regular ritual: I would make a loud announcement to all those sitting in the lobby, "Ladies and gentlemen! Welcome to the famous singer from Spring Street in Kiryat, Shmona," and Diana would shyly smile. She was born in India, and loved to sing songs from her birthplace. Despite her memory deceiving her (often she would forget the names of her children and grandchildren), she remembered many songs, and loved to sing them.

Our ritual was diligently observed through the weeks and months she was hospitalized. After my announcement about the "renowned singer from the north," Diana would always ask me what to sing, and I would always suggest the famous Hindi song, "Ichak dana bichak dana." She would begin to sing in a beautiful, clear voice, a big smile on her face. When she finished singing, I would applaud enthusiastically and signal to the nurses to do the same. Several other patients would join in as well, and Diana would be so happy. The patter between the songs included imaginary stories about the famous singer Diana who had arrived from Hollywood today and who, next week, would be performing in London and Mumbai.

A few days before she died, I arrived at the ward and found her in her chair. "I have no strength to sing today," she said, "I have no air." "No worries," I responded, "just sing in a whisper." Diana sang in a whisper, smiling . . . and that's how I remember her.

In "The Importance of Singing with the Elderly," A. A. Clair says that singing facilitates solace for patients with dementia, provides a consolation in a world which is impossible for them to understand (2000). Song provides an emotional consolation without the need for complicated cognitive processes, and alleviates distress without any connection to vocal quality. Singing also enables the practice of breathing which is beneficial to the patient, helping lift the mood and create an experience of normality as well as enhance self-image. Song creates human contact with others, that of emotional intimacy.

Diana was comforted by her singing. While singing, she looked calmer, and the agitation which gripped her during most of her waking hours subsided. Many cases point out that music has a beneficial effect on the emotional storms of patients with dementia. Singing was Diana's refuge as a normal experience, and she very much enjoyed the attention she received when I announced her as the "famous singer," and when her audience applauded. This contributed to her feeling positive and confident. Several other patients joined in her song, and their singing together reinforced the social bond and the sense of sharing.

Mixed-Up Michael

Michael, 88 years old, had been hospitalized for several months, and his cognitive state was deteriorating. He never remembered his room or his bed and would often slowly walk into the nearest room and lie down in someone else's bed, often putting on spectacles that did not belong to him. Each time I saw him, I would call out to him loudly, ask him how he was, and Michael would answer back just as loudly that his health was excellent. In his youth, he had served as the deputy mayor of his city, could speak seven languages, and was an accountant by profession.

In the early days of our acquaintance, we would dance to the sounds of Turkish songs he loved. He also loved jokes, so I would tell him many, one leading to another, and he would always ask for "just one more." But when his condition began to deteriorate, he no longer remembered the jokes I told him in the past. So I had no need to brainstorm new jokes, since he would laugh at the old ones as if he were hearing them for the first time. He would sit on a chair, staring ahead and looking confused. But when he saw me he would gesture weakly with his hand, as if to say that everything in this world is transient, that we are guests here for a short time. I would mirror his gesture in response, and we would exchange smiles. Later, he would beckon me to come closer and tell him some jokes.

Due to the deterioration in cognitive function, humor, laughter, and smiles are an important element in communicating with patients with dementia, helping them to connect with their environment and improve their overall feeling. For Michael, the jokes were a kind of bridge over the abyss opened up by his illness. The more time passed, and his condition deteriorated, the fewer jokes he remembered. Perhaps he no longer even understood them. Nevertheless, Michael held on to the format of interpersonal communication known as "jokes," as if they were a life preserver. The jokes were a means to communicate with the world through me, and this connection improved his mood. For the jokes themselves, by this stage of his mental deterioration they had no meaning; the meaning lay in the connection we formed through them.

The positive impact of medical clowning on patients with dementia is known, but still not recognized widely. This practice has been associated mainly with clowning for hospitalized children, and much less frequently with older people with dementia or other incurable diseases. Medical clowning can be an important addition to the therapy for patients with dementia, complementing the medical treatment with a holistic approach whose stated goal is caring for the patient's physical and emotional well-being.

It is also effective in working with such patients because it is, by its very nature, an interdisciplinary expressive therapy, integrating several skills such as drama, music, and dance, while conducting a humorous interaction. Each of these arts has a beneficial therapeutic effect on patients with dementia, and the clown's capabilities and skills, together with humor and fantasy, are what enable a unique interaction with so many possibilities.

CHAPTER THIRTEEN

The Future of Medical Clowning

There is a story told about a conference of futurologists held in Paris, around 150 years ago. The participants gathered in an attempt to predict the problems that would engage the city fathers of the future. Their conclusion: the greatest problem would be the horse manure accumulating from the horses pulling the carriages, the city's main mode of transportation. A century and a half later, the horses are gone, replaced by cars. Apparently there are more pressing problems than horse manure to worry the municipal leaders of Paris.

The world changes rapidly. When my children asked me one day what profession I thought they might work at when they were older, I responded that it may not have been invented yet. Take me, for example: when I was a kid, the profession of medical clown did not yet exist but that is my work now. New professions are born out of society's changing needs, innovative technologies, and a changing worldview. Young people must adapt themselves to the constantly changing environment, especially that of the dynamic workplace. The four important forecasting methodologies developed in the 20th-century Delphi, Environmental Scanning, Issues Management and Emerging Issue Analysis, are engaged in predicting global processes and trends and not just examining professions at high resolution. No one in the mid-nineteenth century could have predicted the profession of medical clown or its future.

The historical roots of medical clowning are firmly planted in shamanism and the medieval carnival clowning. Contemporary clown doctors have their inception in the evolved worldview within the Western healthcare system with regard to the place of laughter and humor or, rather, more correctly, the lack of it. Although it was possible to have found clowns in hospitals more than 100 years ago, as shown in the picture published in the Parisian newspaper *Le Petit Journal* in 1908, in which we see two clowns performing for children in a pediatrics ward of a hospital in London, Prof. Atay Citron argues that it was only since the 1960s that Western medicine opened up to alternative and traditional medicine from East Asia, and adopted the approach that humor and laughter are beneficial to health (2011). Prof. Citron, as head of the Department of Theatre, University of Haifa, led the formation of the first full-time academic training program in the world for medical clowns, in collaboration with the Dream Doctors Project, awarding an undergraduate degree in a combined curriculum in interdisciplinary studies and theater.

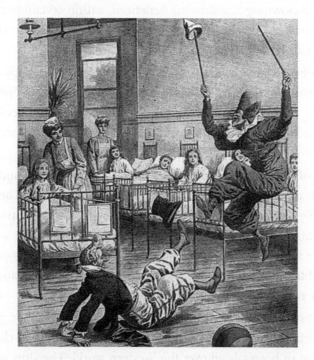

FIGURE 13.1 A front-page illustration and an accompanying report about clowns performing for children in a pediatrics ward in London was published in *Le Petit Journal* (September 1908).

Prof. Citron also shared his thoughts in an interview (on April 2014) I conducted with him, and during which he spoke about the future of medical clowning. According to him, cclowning has not really changed or developed over the past few decades. If we were able to view documentary films of clowns from hundreds of years ago, we would observe that contemporary clowning is not more different or more developed than that of the past. Apparently it will not change very much in the future either.

As for medical clowning, he predicts that it will become officially established as a recognized paramedical profession, and it is fairly certain that medical clowns will be deployed in more and more wards, including adult wards, in hospitals. The more evidence-based scientific studies are conducted showing that medical-clowning assistance is beneficial, within certain parameters, during medical procedures, the more medical clowns will be included in treatment and therapeutic procedures.

In Prof. Citron's view, medical clowning is also an inspiration and point of origin for a re-examination of the issue of "performance" in the hospital—both the doctors' and nurses' performance and that of others in the multidisciplinary care team, and the impact on patients and their recovery processes.

Prof. Citron is not so sure that medical clowning will undergo significant change in the future; it might, however, lead or be part of a re-examination of modern medicine which is so focused on medications and surgical interventions. Western medicine seems to have abandoned, for the most part, aspects that were customary in traditional medicine and associated with performance and the interpersonal relations between healer and patient.

Western medicine has changed its outlook on humor, proof of which are the hundreds (if not thousands) of medical clowns working in hospitals all over the Western world. The story of the pioneer clown doctor, "Patch" Adams, was publicized in the 2000 biopic starring Robin Williams. The film depicted Dr. Hunter Doherty "Patch" Adams's struggle as a medical student against the

Dean of the school, who warned against any human connection with the patients or exhibitions of humor by the medical students in the hospital. The story had a great impact on many medical students throughout the world, including Dr. Assi Cicurel. Dr. Cicurel is an extraordinary physician, living in a rural settlement in the desert and working according as a family doctor deeply involved in community life. He also volunteers every year or two at the Gesundheit Institute founded by Patch Adams in West Virginia.

During an interview with Dr. Cicurel in April 2014, he related the frustration he felt at the technical approach of modern medicine, reflected in the focus on the illness and not on the patient, as well as the limited time devoted to the patient. His first trip to the Gesundheit Institute was in 2005, after he read Patch Adams's book, and attempted medical clowning for the first time. He described medical clowning as a good way to practice bonding with people and the limitless love that physicians have in their work. While at the Gesundheit Institute, Dr. Cicurel and other volunteer doctors formulated a workshop on clowning, love, and compassion, designed for volunteer doctors at the Institute. Dr. Cicurel told me that, strange as it may seem, love and compassion are not in the medical school curriculum. Over the past decade, Dr. Cicurel has taught at the Joyce and Irving Goldman Medical School and the Medical School for International Health in Ben-Gurion University of the Negev. In recent years, he has been doing his best to introduce a course on medical clowning into the medical school curriculum. He feels that such a course has much to contribute to the physicians of the future. It can provide them with the tools for creating warm, human connections which are amusing and better for treating the patients under their care. Over the past two years, he has succeeded in convincing the medical school administration to include a study module on "Theatrical Skills and Medical Clowning versus Language and Cultural Barriers," striving to make medical clowning studies an integral part of physician training. He predicts that, in the future, medical clowning will become an officially recognized paramedical profession.

Medical clowning engages the emotions—not the study of an individual's emotions directed to a better understanding of their source to bring about healing and alleviation of pain, as proposed by psychotherapy. Medical clowning proposes "anti-seriousness" as an alternative to seriousness, by offering a humorous and fantastical perspective which helps reality appear less threatening, even if only for a short while, to those who are ill and in treatment. Medical clowning offers a clownish, friendly, warm relationship to patients hospitalized in an alienated medical center, as well as an alternative interaction to the medical staff who usually maintain a "professional distance."

Several decades have passed since the "birth" of medical clowning in pediatrics wards of public hospitals in the 1980s, yet it is not as accepted as other well-ordered medical and paramedical professions. Many of the medical clowns work on a voluntary basis while the majority of the professional medical clowns receive their salaries through charitable donations. As far as I know, there is no official salaried position for a medical clown in any ministry of health in any country in the world, and it does not seem to me that this situation will change in the foreseeable future, in a world attempting to cope with financial crises and budget cuts by the healthcare system. And yet, this is an irreversible process: medical clowning is now an integral part of pediatrics wards. Much has been written and published about how medical clowns' contribute greatly to improving the emotions and lessen the anxiety of patients. The heads of the healthcare systems in the world have now recognized the importance of the work of medical clowns in the hospital, including the adult wards.

Will there be a breakthrough in the near future in the professional status of the medical clown in terms of having an official salaried position paid for by the hospital budget on a permanent, regular basis? As I see it, recognition will increase as to the necessity of medical clowns, and the demand for their presence in pediatrics and adult wards will increase. This will perhaps generate change in the medical clowns' status in the healthcare system.

Medical clowning established a firm foothold in pediatrics wards, but, due to the abovementioned budgetary constraints, as well as reasons of consciousness, it has remained "stuck" in children's units for many years, while the gerontology and adult departments are crying out for medical clowns. Very few adult wards are lucky enough to have visits by medical clowns. Several nonprofit medical clowning organizations, such as the MiMakkus in the Netherlands, do work with adult patients; but these NGOs are a minority among the vast majority of clown associations working with children. The Dream Doctors Project now has 3 medical clowns who work exclusively with adults out of the more than 70 working in pediatrics wards. When I began working as a medical clown in the adult oncology day unit at Chaim Sheba Medical Center, I encountered a lack of enthusiasm at my presence, expressed by the head nurse. It took her several months to admit that the patients were waiting very impatiently for me to visit, and that my presence in the unit made everyone feel better. A medical clown in adult wards is still not a "given," even though the need is no less than among children. I foresee that this need will receive a proper response, albeit gradually: medical clowns will slowly show an increased presence in adult departments, and their position will not be the first to terminated when budget cuts are being made.

Clowning has been part of human societies since the dawn of time. In previous chapters, I have discussed and compared medical clowns to carnival clowns, shamans, ritual clowns, and clown entertainers (comprising court jesters, circus clowns and street festival clowns). Clowning, in all its multiple forms, varied expressions, and different functions it has fulfilled in human societies has, over the years, undergone a process of evolution and adaptation according to the humanistic needs of the individual and the consensus and narrative of the society in which the clown operates. Stress is one of the outstanding characteristics of life in modern societies—about 50% of the population in the West suffers from hypertension caused by work-related stress. It is interesting to note that hypertension is nonexistent in a society of hunter-gatherers.

A study published by the US National Institute for Occupational Safety and Health found that long work hours cause "acute myocardial infarction, diabetes mellitus, hypertension, subfecundity, and preterm birth" (Caruso et. al. 2004: 28). Tension in the workplace causes not only physical illness but also puts workers at risk of depression or physical pains and chronic fatigue. In a study on tensions at work, it was found that a high percentage of employees pointed to their job as the main stress factor in their lives. The question arises as to whether it is possible to integrate medical clowning as an essential part not only of the hospital but also other areas of our lives—in our workplaces, institutions, and government agencies with whom we citizens have some friction. Actually, we can use clowns in every place which creates tension in us, the tension and stress so characteristic of life in modern society.

EPILOGUE

Prof. Doctor's Story

An Auto-ethnographic Monologue of a Medical Clown Working
with the Terminally Ill

The Epilogue presents the story of my medical clown persona from his viewpoint, in his own words. The fantastic story of his life as he often relates it in the ward. Items from my own curriculum vitae are interwoven with "his" life story, but the other parts of Prof. Doctor's life story have nothing in common with mine. This mixture is the basis for the persona of Prof. Doctor, the Department Head. This mélange is also the infrastructure for the fantasy, humor, and philosophy by means of which he connects with the patients in the Oncology Ward.

And now, introducing the medical clown, Prof. Doctor himself . . . Let's give him the floor. A big hand of applause for the poetical-philosophical monologue by "the medical clown from the Oncology Ward."

Many patients are curious to know more about me, about how I became a medical clown. They want me to tell them my story. And so: I was born into a family of Gypsies. My family wandered with the circus. My acrobat mother was killed in a fall from a high trapeze when I was a toddler, but I have some memories which come to my mind when I think of her. As for my father, I am unable to state with certainty who he actually was, because both the juggler and the dog trainer each claimed passionately that he was my father. Sometimes they would fight about it. At other times they would walk arm in arm, drunkenly reminiscing about their departed lover . . . The patients tend to cast doubts on my life story and my family saga. I also doubt it but as time goes by, memories become elusive for all of us . . .

For many years, before I became a medical clown, I held the (self-appointed) position of the Eternal Clown for Human Existence. As such, the Eternal Clown may not belong to or become a part of life. To be an International Eternal Clown one must, first and foremost, look on from the side without belonging to a specific place, time, and society. The Eternal Clown must see-all and be-all in perpetual motion, hear all and continue touching upon the lives of all who encounter him, laugh with them, then bid them farewell. The Eternal Clown is an onlooker. He experiences the comradeship of a moment shared in this tortured/painful place . . . This is similar to my current work in the Oncology Ward where I travel through cities, villages, and countries.

I slept in the street, in store rooms, in bedrooms of one-night lovers, on the beachfront, in vacant student housing, at the houses of new friends who became old friends over the years. I saw the surprised face of a Gypsy thief from the Triana quarter in Seville as he shattered the windscreen of my car in the middle of the night, and saw my no-less-surprised face . . . I played flamenco guitar with the Gypsies . . . saw an Italian lad juggle nine balls on the sidewalk, and watched a Dutch guy fall from a trapeze, face-down. I saw a man draw a knife on his sweetheart . . . I've lived in a prostitute's house in Amsterdam's "red light" district . . . I've built a unicycle from an old bicycle with clowns and acrobats from a commune in Belgium. A woman and her elderly father gathered me up into their home to save me from having to sleep under a bridge with all of the clochards. I saw all those who sit in the coffee houses in the village squares, the families in the park, the homeless drunkards freezing out on the benches.

I have received improper suggestions. People have tried to cheat me, fool me, help me, love me, hurt me, and ignore me. They teased me and laughed at my clown attire. They helped me repair my car in the name of brotherhood, and invited me into their homes for fraternity's sake, into their beds for the love of passion, they asked me to remain in the name of love. I saw them alive, I saw the blink of an eye and I saw everything. I have been witness to suffering, evil, routine, goodness, foolishness, love, and the story of my life—which may or may not have been lived . . . In the Oncology Ward I sometimes hear life stories from people on their deathbed, grasping at the words such as "a passing dream," illusory life stories just like my own curriculum vitae.

I purchased a guitar form the Gypsies of Seville and learned from them how to strum a tempestuous flamenco, the Bolero, and Algerian rais. When I busked in the streets, people threw coins and hashish into my upturned hat . . . When I play my guitar in the Oncology Ward, the patients with the IV lines in their arms, receiving their chemotherapy, dance their fingers to the rhythm of the flamenco, and when I raise my husky voice in song—as befits a flamenco singer of dirges, who usually sound hoarse—the patients offer to share their medicinal marijuana with me.

In the corner cafe I met curly-haired Maria Rossa, the Gypsy, the stunning waitress, as lovely as Carmen in Carlos Saura's film. When I describe to the patients how she taught me elementary Spanish amid orgasmic moans, they erupt with laughter until they are breathless.

At the Bannhofstrasse in Zurich, Switzerland, in front of the great banks, I played with my lover the flautist, the one who taught me how to play jazz. Once I played "What a Wonderful World" to a dying patient, imitating Louis Armstrong's hoarse voice. He smiled a final smile and bid farewell to me with his eyes . . .

At the Pompidou Center, among the fakirs who "hang out" there, lying on their beds of nails, eating glass, I threw the diablo up to the skies and rode a tall unicycle. I can speak French gibberish very, very fast—entirely unintelligible, a skill that a not-inconsiderable number of patients found very amusing . . .

Italian Border Police, on the border with France, asked me to perform for them, to juggle balls and clubs. They closed the crossing for several minutes just to enjoy the show. Because of this memory, I like to dress up at times as an Italian policeman and to walk like a duck through the Oncology Ward, marching to a martial rhythm (with my right hand and leg moving together, as well as the left limbs moving in coordination with each other) while singing the famous revolutionary song:

Avanti o popolo, allariscossa,
Bandierarossa, Bandierarossa
Avanti o popolo, allariscossa,
Bandierarossa trionferà.

Bandierarossa la trionferà
Bandierarossa la trionferà
Bandierarossa la trionferà
Evvivailcomunismo e la libertà

One of the nurses is a good friend of mine; she joins me in song and marches behind me; we walk in a line like a pair of police officers as we salute the patients.

Once, a patient who was terminally ill, presented me with his autobiography, a book he wrote about his childhood and the special relationship with his mother. The next day, I arrived at the ward with the following dialogue, which I'd written, and which I read aloud to him:

Mother. O my sweet boy, you'll be entering this world in a few moments, which will change the universe for ever.

Son. It didn't change at all when I emerged from your womb, Mother . . . and it won't change a bit when I disappear . . . I'm cold, Mom . . . hug me . . .

Mother. I'll hug you even when you're wet and writhing. Just cry, your little voice will announce to the world that you're here.

Son. Mom, where are you at my last moments? Where's your warm palm that knows how to caress so well, how to calm me down . . .

Mother. The only chick-like scent that will waft toward my nose . . . I will draw it close to me, precious soul . . . apple of my eye . . . my little loved one . . .

Son. Oh my god . . . Hey! I see God . . . that's strange, oh my goodness, He looks just the way I imagined him when I was young, with a long, white beard, and . . . He's sailing on a white cloud . . . He's winking to me, I don't believe this, He's signaling to me to come closer . . . I have to ask Him a few things, I'd like him to clear some things up, for example: What's all this about?

Mother. Life awaits you, little son of mine. The world awaits you patiently. Life calls out to you, my sweet one . . . The world is open and wide, you'll grow up and life will smile upon you . . . After all, you're the promise, and life will keep it.

Son: I wasn't the promise, or maybe I was, but life didn't keep its promise.

Mother: You'll be taking the beauty and goodness from life, to their utmost . . . Look, I can see you growing up, I can see you on the swing in kindergarten. Now I see you swimming like a fish, having fun in the waves . . . and your first love . . . who's that beautiful girl who captured your heart?

Son. Hold it a sec, Mom. God is explaining something to me . . . OMG I don't believe it! Mom, I can't believe it, you'll die when you hear this! God is sitting here with me and explaining everything to me. And he has the time, no kidding!

Mother. Run, my boy, go forth into life . . . don't stop. Life will keep its promise. After all, you are the promise . . .

Son. Give me your caressing hand, Mom, it's terribly hard to say goodbye . . . no kidding, it's just like in the stories . . .

I can see a bright white light and snowy mountain peaks . . . I can see myself detaching from my body . . . OMG, it's really true, all the nonsense I heard . . . who woulda' believed it . . . Mom, I have to go . . . I'm going . . . Mom, I'm crazy about you . . . I'll be back in a minute to say goodbye to you . . .

I'll be back right away to say goodbye to life . . . I have to go now. I'm coming back right away to say goodbye . . .

When I finished reading, we looked deeply into each other's eyes in silence and held hands.

I know that when my soul goes "up there" to meet with the Big Red Nose, and is asked to give an account of the many years I spent "down here", I'll relate everything that these eyes have witnessed. My testimony will be recorded by the Lady Clown of the Higher World, with whom I will fall immediately in love. And that will be the conclusion of my part in the great Tikkun Olam Project of Repairing the World. It will be no short testimony, but Lady Clown of the Higher World will have all the patience in the world to write my history down on the feathery clouds. She will write everything I say about the children I met in the various hospital units, about the laughter, the smiles and the dreams. For example, about the dream in which I was standing or, more correctly, hovering, thanks to a pair of huge, amazing white wings which sprouted from my back. There were beds all around, and children lying in the beds. They also had wings on their backs, as did the medical staff in their white smocks. Even the cleaning lady was flying around with her wings, followed by the squeegee and the bucket on smaller wings . . . The Lady Clown will continue to record as I dictate a short eulogy I'll compose about myself: *I'm so sorry about myself. My life has finished, it's ended, it's wasted, gone for good. There will be no more sunsets, nor hot soup during winter. No more kind words, caresses, good jokes, little farts under the blanket, or swims in clear blue waters.* I think that, in the future, I'm going to compose a tune to this eulogy, then sing it in the Hospice. It can become a real hit there!

Sometimes I come to the ward dressed in my beloved Sophia's wedding dress. Sophia, the most beautiful woman in the world, whose beauty and goodness of heart made me fall in love with her. We were married in the small city hall in a village near Naples. Sophia wore a white dress, and I was in an old suit of her father's into which I could barely fit. From Napoli and the southern Italian villages, members of Sophia's wide-branching family descended upon us, male and female cousins overflowing the hall and the courtyard, constantly chattering. I quickly found an apartment in Naples, in an attic on the top floor on Mazcanone Street, very close to the university. It was a teeny tiny apartment, our one and a half rooms in an attic, but we were gloriously happy. Sophia found work in the adjacent restaurant. I would wait for her shift to end, so we could stroll toward the harbor, passing the Piazza del Municipio and the Castelnuovo toward the sea and Via Partenope. We would walk along, gazing at the azure sea and the distant mountains of the bay, at the ships making their way to port, and at the blue skies. We would fill our lungs with the tangy salt air and kiss each other— kisses sweet and looong. In the evenings when we didn't feel like staying in, we would sit in our favorite small cafe on Via Cristoforo Columbo, facing the port. We traveled to Torino and hiked high up along the Via Antigniano, looking down at all the blue spread out beneath us in a dreamy sight. Together we would sing:

> *Volare, oh oh,*
> *Cantare, oh ohohoh.*
> *Nelbludipinto di blu,*
> *felice di stare lassù . . .*

When I arrive at the ward with Sophia's white bridal gown, I stand near the patient's chair as we set sail in my gondola. I take my long oar, push the gondola, and burst out in song; the patient usually joins me. But sometimes, dressed in Sophia's white gown, my feet tap out bridal dances from faraway Yemen, and as I dance

I place kisses on the bald pates of the surprised and amused patients in their armchairs, connected to their chemotherapy infusions. At other times, I dance to music from distant exotic lands, or simply sit down near a patient and embrace her.

At times, I simply stand in the Oncology Ward and listen to the patients' monologues, without jumping or dancing or singing, but only listening attentively. For example, an elderly woman, in a weak voice, told me about her life, of her years of young womanhood, her excitement at falling in love. She spoke of the whirring of the sewing machine, of the fall foliage in a faraway country. Of the children wading in the water, of cigarette smoke drawn into the lungs, of *kapusta*—the delicious dish of stuffed cabbage her mother taught her how to cook before the war. She brought up memories of "that war," in her heavy Hungarian-accented broken Hebrew, albums of yellowing photographs, conversations with her next-door neighbor across the balcony, the warmth of the summer sun heating up the roof, the winter moisture and the rain pounding that same roof. And more . . . holidays and family dinners, with their many dishes, laundry, children bustling about the house and creating a din, the quiet of the nighttime, bedroom games, passion, fatigue, illness, longing, concern, thoughts . . . and still more, about family celebrations, weddings, circumcision feasts, gossip, jealousy, hatred, funerals, farewells, yearning for parents no longer in this world, missing a departed sister, small talk among best friends, telephone calls from children, songs around the Seder table on Passover eve, and songs from a good operetta. She whispered of dreams, of forgetting, old age, illness, the pain, the hospital, the caregivers, visits from grandchildren and the body's final betrayal . . .

After such monologues, I become a thoughtful, contemplative clown. I walk over to a quiet place and I take a deep breath. Engraved in my memory, which melts away as the years go by—two generations after someone has passed, it seems as if he never was. What remains? Descendants, a house which was built, an inheritance to bequeath, money, objects collected over the years most of which are not needed, objects heaped up in the storage space and then thrown into the trash. Perhaps some sort of intellectual property, some creative production, some original plays, a sculpture, paintings, invention, laws passed by the national legislature, legal precedents—these are the things that carry our spirit onward to generations to come. Seasonal spirits, annual spirits, the winds of change, Eastern winds that blow hot and dry out a person's soul . . . Winds bringing much-needed rain, tornados uprooting people and cultures from their homes into concentration camps. Fierce monsoons, and refreshing gentle breezes of twilight. Once we got up in the morning, went walking, built, loved, gave birth to children, feared, created, wrote, and then finally gave up the ghost. Now our curriculum vitae are borne on the winds. Souls bond to similar souls. Ancient souls arising from ancient times hover over the Deep and above the Earth long after the memories of our faces and names have dissolved like clouds scattered by the winds.

After several seconds of deep thought, I blow out a stream of air from my lips (making a sound like a long fart), give myself a little shake, and then get up to dance and sing in the next room. I sing of my beloved Sina from Copenhagen, with whom I sailed away, madly in love, like Vikings embarking in their mighty ships. That took place on the luxurious waterbed in her room. But I became seasick and we had to descend to the safe shore of the carpet. Later, I sang about a beauteous young woman from Isla Bom Jesus dos Passos, whom I met in Bahia, Brazil and with whom we set sail on an old fishing boat and rowed toward the bay where we could gaze at the wonderful sunsets in Bahia de Todosos Santos.

When I arrive at the children's ward, it's another story altogether. There I battle with tiny opponents using my spongy swords, in difficult and vocal battles complete with loud sound effects of warfare. One little kid pursued me with a drawn sword (made out of foam rubber), as I fled like a coward, making loud soldier-like noises, hitting out with my own sword at everyone I encountered along my flight. Finally, I collapsed in a huge drama, taking a very, very long time to "die." My bitter enemy, the short opponent in the battle, strut down the corridor crying out, "Nurse! Nurse! Quick— the clown is dying." Later he came in and saw me open one eye, whereupon the battle recommenced . . . from the beginning . . .

A List of Sources

Some chapters in this volume are edited versions of articles that were originally published elsewhere:

Chapter 1: *TDR* 56(2) (2012): 169–77.

Chapter 3: *Journal of Dramatherapy* 36(1) (2014): 18–26.

Chapter 4: *Journal of Social Semiotics* 24(5) (2014): 599–607.

Chapter 5: *Israeli Journal of Humor Research* 1(4) (2013): 95–111.

Chapter 12: *Journal of Holistic Nursing* 32(3) (2014): 226–31.

References

ACHTERBERG, Jeanne. 1987. "The Shaman: Master Healer in the Imaginary Realm" in Shirley Nicholson (ed.), *Shamanism: An Expanded View of Reality*. Wheaton, IL: Theosophical Publishing House, pp. 103–24.

ALKEMA, Karen, Jeremy M. Linton, and Randall Davies. 2008. "A Study of the Relationship between Self-Care, Compassion Satisfaction, Compassion Fatigue, and Burnout Among Hospice Professionals." *Journal of Social Work in End-Of-Life and Palliative Care* 4(2): 101–19.

AMIR, Lydia. 2012. "He Who Laughs Properly: The Comic in the History of Philosophy" in Arie Sover and Avner Ziv (eds), *The Importance of not Being Serious: A Collection of Multi-Disciplinary Articles in Humor Research*, Hebrew EDN. Jerusalem: Carmel.

ATWAL, Anita, and Kay Caldwell. 2006. "Nurses' Perceptions of Multidisciplinary Team Work in Acute Health-Care." *International Journal of Nursing Practice* 12(6): 359–65.

AYALON, Offra, and Molly Lahad. 1990. *Hayim al hagevul: Hison vehitmodedot bematsavey lahats vesiconim bithonim* [Living on the Border: Strengthening Resilience and Coping with Stress from Security Violence and Risk]. Haifa: Nord/IDF Home Front Command.

BAKHTIN, Mikhail M. 1978a. *Problems of Dostoevsky's Poetics* (Caryl Emerson trans.). Ann Arbor: University of Michigan Press.

———. 1978b. *Sugiyot hapoetika shel Dostoevsky (Problems of Dostoevsky's Poetics)*. Tel Aviv: Sifriat Hapoalim. [Hebrew].

———. 1984. *Rabelais and his World* (Helene Iswolsky trans.). Bloomington, IN: Indiana University Press.

BALA, Michael. 2010. "The Clown: An Archetypal Self-Journey." *Jung Journal: Culture and Psyche* 4(1): 50–71.

BALLARD, Clive G., John O'Brien, Ian James, and Alan Swann (eds). 2001. *Dementia: Management of Behavioral and Psychological Symptoms*. Oxford: Oxford University Press.

BARKER, Larry L. 1971. *Listening Behavior*. Englewood NJ: Prentice-Hall.

BAUDOUIN, Charles. 2015 [1920]. *Suggestion and Autosuggestion: A Psychological and Pedagogical Study Based Upon the Investigation made by the New Nancy School* (Eden and Cedar Paul trans). London: Routledge.

BAUDRILLARD, Jean. 1994. *Simulacra and Simulation* (Sheila Faria Glaser trans.). Ann Arbor: University of Michigan Press.

BENSON, Jill, and Karen Magraith. 2005. "Compassion Fatigue and Burnout: The Role of Balint Groups." *Australian Family Physician* 34(6): 497–8.

BRESSLER, Eric. R., and Sigal Balshine. 2006."The Influence of Humor on Desirability." *Evolution and Human Behavior* 27(1): 29–39.

BROOK, Peter. 1991. *The Empty Space*. London: Penguin.

BUCKWALTER, Kathleen C., Linda. A. Gerdner, Gretchen. R. Hall, John. M. Stolley, P. Kudart, and Shannon Ridgeway. 1995. "Shining Through: The Humour and Individuality of Persons with Alzheimer's Disease." *Journal of Gerontological Nursing* 21(3): 11–16

BUFFUM, Martha D., and Meryl Brod. 1998. "Humor and Well-Being in Spouse Caregivers of Patients with Alzheimer's Disease." *Applied Nursing Research* 11(1): 12–18.

CARP, Cheryl E. 1998. "Clown Therapy: The Creation of a Clown Character as a Treatment Intervention." *Arts in Psychotherapy* 25(4): 245–55.

CARUSO, Claire C., Edward M. Hitchcock, Robert B. Dick, John M. Russo and Jennifer M. Schmit. 2004. "Overtime and Extended Work Shifts: Recent Findings on Illnesses, Injuries, and Health Behaviors." Cincinnati, OH: NIOSH Publications Dissemination.

CITRON, Atay. 2011. "Medical Clowning and Performance Theory" in James Harding and Cindy Rosenthal (eds), *The Rise of Performance Studies: Rethinking Richard Schechner's Broad Spectrum*. London: Palgrave Macmillan, pp. 248–63.

CLAIR, Alicia A. 2000. "The Importance of Singing with Elderly Patients" in David Aldridge (ed.), *Music Therapy in Dementia Care*. London: Jessica Kingsley Publishers, pp. 81–101.

CLARK, Michael E., Anne W. Lipe and Melinda Bilbrey. 1998. "Use of Music to Decrease Aggressive Behaviors in People with Dementia." *Journal of Gerontological Nursing* 27(7): 10–17.

CLAUW, Daniel. J., and David. A. Williams. 2002. "Relationship Between Stress and Pain in Work-related Upper Extremity Disorders: The

Hidden Role of Chronic Multisymptom Illnesses." *American Journal Industrial Medicine* 41: 370–82.

COOKE, Nancy J., Eduardo Salas, Preston A. Kiekel, and Brian Bell. 2004. "Advances in Measuring Team Cognition" in Eduardo Salas and Stephen M. Fiore (eds), *Team Cognition: Understanding the Factors That Drive Process and Performance*. Washington, DC: American Psychological Association, pp. 83–106.

BASTING, Anne D. 2001. "'God Is a Talking Horse': Dementia and Performance of Self." *TDR* 45(3): 78–94.

DAVIS, Mark H. 1994. *Empathy: A Social Psychological Approach*. Madison, WI: Brown and Benchmark.

DREAM DOCTORS PROJECT. 2009. *Rofei Hahalom* [The Dream Doctors: Clowns in the Service of Medicine]. Philnor Foundation. Available on YouTube: https://goo.gl/bFLA3p (last accessed on July 30, 2017).

DU BOIS-REYMOND, Manuela. 1998. "'I Don't Want to Commit Myself Yet': Young People's Life Concepts." *Journal of Youth Studies* 1(1): 63–79.

DUIGNAN, Debbie, Lynne Hedley, and Rachael Milverton. 2009. "Exploring Dance as a Therapy for Symptoms and Social Interaction in Dementia." *Nursing Times* 105(30): 19–22.

ERICKSON, Milton H. 1980. *The Nature of Hypnosis and Suggestion*. New York: Irvington.

EVANS-PRITCHARD, Edward Evan. 1976. *Witchcraft, Oracles, and Magic Among the Azande*. Oxford: Clarendon Press.

EYER, Joseph. 1975. "Hypertension as a Disease of Modern Society." *International Journal of Health Services* 5(4): 539–58.

FISKE, John. 1990. *Introduction to Communication Studies*. London: Routledge.

———. 1989a. *Understanding Popular Culture*, 2nd EDN. London: Routledge.

———. 1989b. "Offensive Bodies and Carnival Pleasures" in *Understanding Popular Culture*, 2nd EDN. London: Routledge, pp. 56–82.

FOUCAULT, Michel. 1975. *Discipline and Punish: The Birth of the Prison* (Alan Sheridan trans.). New York: Random House

———. 2003. *The Birth of the Clinic*. London: Routledge.

FRIEDLER, Shevach, Saralee Glasser, Liat Azani, Laurence S. Freedman, Arie Raziel, Dvora Strassburger, Raphael Ron-El, and Liat

Lerner-Geva. 2011. "The Effect of Medical Clowning on Pregnancy Rates After In Vitro Fertilization Embryo Transfer." *Fertility and Sterility* 95(6): 2127–30.

GELKOPF, Marc. 2011. "The Use of Humor in Serious Mental Illness: A Review." *Evidence-Based Complementary and Alternative Medicine*: 1–8.

GERVAIS, Nicole, Bernie Warren, and Peter Twohig. 2006. "Nothing Seems Funny Anymore: Studying Burnout in Clown Doctors" in Aubrey D. Litvack (ed.), *Making Sense of: Stress, Humour and Healing*. Oxford: Inter-Disciplinary Press, pp. 77–82. Available at: https://goo.gl/cJSHmJ (last accessed on July 30, 2017).

GLASPER, Edward A., Gill Prudhoe, and Katie Weaver. 2007. "Does Clowning Benefit Children in Hospital?: Views of Theodora Children's Trust Clown Doctors." *Journal of Children's and Young People's Nursing* 1(1): 24–8.

GOLAN, G., P. Tighe, N. Dobija, A. Perel, and I. Keidan. 2009. "Clowns for the Prevention of Preoperative Anxiety in Children: A Randomized Controlled Trial." *Pediatric Anesthesia* 19(3): 262–66.

GRINBERG, Zohar, Susana Pendzik, Ronen Kowalsky, and Yaron "Sancho" Goshen. 2012. "Drama Therapy Role Theory as A Context for Understanding Medical Clowning." *Arts in Psychotherapy* (39)1: 42–51. Available at: https://goo.gl/xQcHMD (last accessed on July 30, 2017).

HANDELMAN, Don. 1990. *Models and Mirrors: Towards an Anthropology of Public Events*. Cambridge: Cambridge University Press.

———. 1981. "The Ritual Clown: Attributes and Affinities." *Anthropos* 76: 321–68.

HANSEN, Lars K., Maria Kibaek, Torben Martinussen, Lene Kragh, and Mogens Hejl. 2011. "Effect of a Clown's Presence at Botulinum Toxin Injections in Children: A Randomized Prospective Study." *Journal of Pain Research* 4: 297–300.

HARMAN, Guy, and Clare Linda. 2006. "Illness Representations and Lived Experience in Early-Stage Dementia." *Qualitative Health Research* 16(4): 484–502.

HARNER, Michael. 1990. *The Way of the Shaman*. San Francisco, CA: Harper and Row.

———, and Gary Doore. 1987. "The Ancient Wisdom in Shamanic Cultures" in Shirley J. Nicholson (ed.), *Shamanism: An Expanded View of Reality*. Wheaton, IL: Theosophical Publishing House, pp. 3–16.

HENDRIKS, Ruud. 2012. "Tackling Indifference—Clowning, Dementia, and the Articulation of a Sensitive Body." *Medical Anthropology: Cross-Cultural Studies in Health and Illness* 31(6): 459–76.

JACQUES, A., and G. Jackson. 2000. *Understanding Dementia*, 3rd EDN. Edinburgh: Churchill Livingstone.

KATZ, Robert L. 1963. *Empathy: Its Nature and Uses*. New York: Free Press of Glencoe/Crowell-Collier.

KAYE, Nick. 2000. *Site-Specific Art: Performance, Place and Documentation*. London: Routledge.

KITWOOD, T. 1997. "The Experience of Dementia." *Aging and Mental Health* 1(1): 13–22.

KLEIN, Allen. 1989. *The Healing Power of Humor: Techniques for Getting Through Loss, Setbacks, Upsets, Disappointments, Difficulties, Trials, Tribulations, and All that Not-so-funny Stuff*. New York: Jeremy P. Tarcher/Putnam.

———. 1998. *The Courage to Laugh*. New York: Tarcher/Putnam

KOLLER, Donna, and Camilla Gryski. 2008. "The Life Threatened Child and the Life Enhancing Clown: Towards a Model of Therapeutic Clowning." *Evidence Based Complementary Alternative Medicine* 5(1): 17–25.

KROGER, Susan M., Kathryn Chapin, and Melissa Brotons. 1999. "Is Music Therapy an Effective Intervention for Dementia? A Meta-Analytic Review of Literature." *Journal of Music Therapy* 36(1): 2–15.

KWON, Miwon. 2004. *One Place After Another: Site-Specific Art and Locational Identity*. Cambridge, MA: MIT Press.

LAHAD, Mooli. 1992. "Story-making in Assessment Method for Coping with Stress: Six-piece Story-making and BASIC Ph" in Sue Jennings (ed.), *Dramatherapy: Theory and Practice*, VOL. 2. London: Routledge, pp. 150–63.

LANG, Trudi. 1995. "An Overview of Four Futures Methodologies." *Manoa Journal* 7: 1–43.

LINGE, Lotta. 2011. "Joy Without Demands: Hospital Clowns in The World of Ailing Children." *International Journal of Qualitative Studies Health Well-being* 6(1): 10.

LOHFF, Brigitte. 2001. "Self-Healing Forces and Concepts of Health and Disease: A Historical Discourse." *Theoretical Medicine and Bioethics* 22(6): 543–64.

Luquette, John. 2007. "Stress, Compassion Fatigue, Burnout: Effective Self-care Techniques for Oncology Nurses." *Oncology Nursing Forum* 34(2): 490.

Manor-Binyamini, Iris. 2009. *Multidisciplinary Teamwork: Theory, Research and Application,* Hebrew EDN. Jerusalem: Ministry of Education.

Mathews, Richard. 2002. *The Liberation of Imagination.* London: Routledge.

McCallin, A., and A. Bamford. 2007. "Interdisciplinary Teamwork: Is the Influence of Emotional Intelligence Fully Appreciated?" *Journal of Nursing Management* 15(4): 386–91.

McFadden, Susan H. 2004. "The Paradoxes of Humor and the Burdens of Despair." *Journal of Religious Gerontology* 16 (3–4): 13–27.

McGhee, Paul. 2010. *Humor: the Lighter Path to Resilience and Health.* Bloomington, IN: Authorhouse.

Menzies, Heather. 2005. *No Time: Stress and Crisis of Modern Life.* Vancouver: Douglas and McIntyre.

Meyer, John. C. 2000. "Humour as a Double-Edged Sword: Four Functions of Humour in Communication." *Communication Theory* 10(3): 310–31.

Monroe, S. M. 2008. "Modern Approaches to Conceptualizing and Measuring Human Life Stress." *Annual Review of Clinical Psychology* 4: 33–52

Montgomery, Guy H., Katherine N. Duhamel, and William H. Redd. 2008. "A Meta-Analysis of Hypnotically Induced Analgesia: How Effective Is Hypnosis?" *International Journal of Clinical and Experimental Hypnosis* 48(2): 138–53.

Moody Jr., Raymond A. 1978. *Laugh after Laugh: The Healing Power of Humor.* Jacksonville, FL: Headwaters Press.

Nancarrow, Susan A., Andrew Booth, Steven Ariss, Tony Smith, Pam Enderby, and Alison Roots. 2013. "Ten Principles of Good Interdisciplinary Team Work." *Human Resources for Health* 11: 19. Available at: https://goo.gl/Wo7th (last accessed on July 30, 2017).

Nevo, Roth. 1984. *Hakomedia hashakespearit* [Shakespearean Comedy]. Jerusalem: Keter. [Hebrew].

Nilsson, U., N. Rawal, L. E. Unestahl, C. Zetterberg, and M. Unosson. 2001. "Improved Recovery After Music and Therapeutic Suggestions During General Anaesthesia: A Double-Blind Randomised Controlled Trial." *Acta Anaesthesiologica Scandinavica* 45(7): 812–17.

NUTTMAN-SHWARTZ, Orit, Rachel Scheyer, and Herzl Tzioni. 2010. "Medical Clowning: Even Adults Deserve a Dream." *Social Work in Health Care* 49(6): 581–98.

OSTROWER, Chaya. 2009. *Lelo humor hayino mitabdim* (If Not for Humor, We Would Have Committed Suicide). Israel: Yad Vashem. [Hebrew].

PALO-BENGTSSON, Liisa, and Sirkka-Liisa Ekman. 2000. "Dance Events as a Caregiver Intervention for Persons with Dementia." *Nursing Inquiry* 7(3): 156–65.

PENDZIK Susana, and Amnon Raviv. 2011. "Therapeutic Clowning and Drama Therapy: A family resemblance." *Arts in Psychotherapy* 38(4): 267–75.

PLESTER, Barbara, and Mark Orams. 2008. "Send in the Clowns: The Role of the Joker in Three New Zealand IT Companies." *Humor* 21(3): 253–81

PUETZ, Babette. 2007 [2003]. *The Symposium and Komos in Aristophanes*, 2nd EDN. Oxford: Aris and Phillips.

RAVIV, Amnon. 2012a. "Still the Best Medicine Even in A War Zone: My Work as a Medical Clown." *TDR* 56(4): 169–77.

———. 2012b. "The Clown Doctor in Emergency: Theory and Practice" in Avner Ziv and Arie Sover (eds), *The Importance of Not Being Serious: Collection of Multidisciplinary Articles in Humor Research*, Hebrew EDN. Jerusalem: Carmel, pp. 318–30.

RENTSCH, Joan R., and David. J. Woehr. 2004. "Quantifying Congruence in Cognition: Social Relations Modeling and Team Member Schema Similarity" in Eduardo Salas and S. M. Fiore (eds), *Team Cognition: Understanding the Factors that Drive Process and Performance*. Washington: American Psychological Association, pp. 11–31.

ROBINSON, Vera M. 1991. *Humor and the Health Professions: The Therapeutic Use of Humor in Health Care*. Thorofare, NJ: Slack.

ROURKE, Mary T. 2007. "Compassion Fatigue in Pediatric Palliative Care Providers." *Pediatric Clinics of North America* 54(5): 631–44.

RUSSELL, Daniel. 2005. *Plato on Pleasure and the Good Life*. Oxford: Clarendon Press.

SALAS, Eduardo, Michael A. Rosen, Shawn C. Burke, and Gerald F. Goodwin. 2009. "The Wisdom Of Collective In Organization: An Update Of The Team Work Competence" in Eduardo Salas, G. F.

Goodwin, and C. S. Burke (eds), *Team Effectiveness in Complex Organizations: Cross Disciplinary Perspectives and Approaches*. New York: Taylor and Francis, pp. 39–55.

SAUNDERS, Pamela. 1998. "'You're Out of Your Mind!': Humor as a Face-Saving Strategy During Neuropsychological Examinations." *Health Communication* 10 (4), 357–72.

SCHECHNER, Richard. 1993. *The Future of the Rituals: Writing on Culture and Performance*. Oxon: Routledge.

—————. 2002. *Performance Studies: An Introduction*, 2nd EDN. New York: Routledge.

—————, and Willa Appel (eds). 1990. *By Means of Performance: Intercultural Studies of Theatre and Ritual*. Cambridge: Cambridge University Press.

SCHEFF, Thomas. J. 1979. *Catharsis in Healing, Ritual, and Drama*. Berkeley: University of California Press.

SEHGAL, Niraj L., Michael Fox, Arpana R. Vidyarthi, Bradley A. Sharpe, Susan Gearhart, Thomas Bookwalter, Jack Barker, Brian K. Alldredge, Mary A. Blegen, and Robert M. Wachter. 2008. "A Multidisciplinary Teamwork Training Program: The Triad for Optimal Patient Safety (TOPS) Experience." *Journal of General Internal Medicine* 23(12): 2053–7.

SENGE, Peter M. 1990. *The Fifth Discipline: The Art and Practice of the Learning Organization*. New York: Doubleday/Currency.

SHANI, Nimrod. 1998. *Mehkar Phenomenologia shel havayot hahitmasrut lahavaya* (A Phenomenological Study of Experiences of Letting Go). Ramat Aviv, Israel: Bar Ilan University. [Hebrew].

SHEA, J. D. C. 1991. "Suggestion, Placebo, and Expectation: Immune Effects and Other Bodily Change" in J. F. Schumaker (ed.) *Human Suggestibility: Advances in Theory, Research, and Application*. New York: Routledge, pp. 253–76.

SHOSTAK, Marjorie . 1981. *Nisa: The Life and Words of a !kung Woman*. London: Allen Lane.

SPIELBERGER, C. D. 2010. "Job Stress Survey" in I. B. Weiner and W. E. Craighead (eds), *Corsini Encyclopedia of Psychology*, VOL. 1, 4th EDN. Hoboken, NJ: John Wiley and Sons.

SPITZER, Peter. 2006. "Laughter Boss" in Aubrey D. Litvack (ed.), *Making Sense of Stress, Humour and Healing*. Oxford: Inter-Disciplinary Press, pp. 83–5. Available at: https://goo.gl/dsxnux (last accessed on July 30, 2017).

————. 2011. "The LaughterBoss™" in Hilary Lee and Trevor Adams (eds), *Creative Approaches in Dementia Care*. New York: Palgrave Macmillan, pp. 32–53.

STEVENS, John. 2012. "Stand Up for Dementia: Performance, Improvisation and Stand Up Comedy as Therapy for People with Dementia: A Qualitative Study." *Dementia* 11(1): 61–73.

STOUGH, Con, Donald Saklofske, and James Parker (eds). 2009. *Assessing Emotional Intelligence: Theory, Research, and Applications*. New York: Springer.

SUNG, Huei-Chuan, Shu-Min Chang, Wen-li Lee, and Ming-shinn Lee. 2006. "The Effects of Group Music with Movement Intervention on Agitated Behaviours of Institutionalized Elders with Dementia in Taiwan." *Complementary Therapies in Medicine* 14(2): 113–19.

TAKEDA, Masatoshi, Ryota Hashimoto, Takashi Kudo, Masayasu Okochi, Shinji Tagami, Takashi Morihara, Golam Sadick, and Toshihisa Tanaka. 2010. "Laughter and Humor as Complementary and Alternative Medicines for Dementia Patients." *BMC Complementary and Alternative Medicine* 10: 28.

TENER, Dafna, Rachel Lev-Wiesel, Nessia Lang Franco, and Shoshi Ofir. 2010. "Laughing Through This Pain: Medical Clowning During Examination of Sexually Abused Children—An Innovative Approach." *Journal of Child Sexual Abuse* 19: 128–40.

TURNER, Victor W. 1969. *The Ritual Process: Structure and Anti-structure*. Chicago: Aldine.

VAGNOLI, Laura, Simona Caprilli, Arianna Robiglio and Andrea Messeri. 2005. "Clown Doctors as a Treatment for Preoperative Anxiety in Children: A Randomized, Prospective Study." *Pediatrics* 116(4): 563–67.

VAN BLERKOM, Linda Miller. 1995. "Clown Doctors: Shaman Healers of Western Medicine." *Medical Anthropology Quarterly* 9 (4): 462–75.

VIOLETS, Marion. 2000. "'We'll Survive': An Experiential View of Dance Movement Therapy for People with Dementia" in David Aldridge (ed.), *Music Therapy in Dementia Care*. London: Jessica Kingsley, pp. 212–28.

WANG, Jianli. 2005. "Work Stress as a Risk Factor for Major Depressive Episode(s)." *Psychological Medicine*: 865–71.

WEE, David, and Diane Myers. 2003. "Compassion Satisfaction, Compassion Fatigue, and Critical Incident Stress Management." *International Journal of Emergency Mental Health* 5(1): 33–7.

WINKELMAN, Michael. 2010. *Shamanism: A Biopsychosocial Paradigm of consciousness and Healing.* California: ABC-CLIO.

XYRICHIS, A., and E. Ream. 2008. "Teamwork: A Concept Analysis." *Journal of Advanced Nursing* 61(2): 232–41.